Bayesian Approaches in Oncology Using R and OpenBUGS

Bayesian Approaches in Oncology Using R and OpenBUGS

Atanu Bhattacharjee

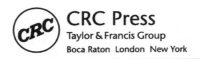

CRC Press
Taylor & Francis Group
Boca Raton London New York

CRC Press is an imprint of the
Taylor & Francis Group, an **informa** business
A CHAPMAN & HALL BOOK

I dedicated this book to Dr.Balekudaru Shantha, Ophthalmologist, Director, Sankara Nethralaya Chennai, for preserving my vision in a critical time.

Contents

Preface   xiii

Author   xv

I   Bayesian in Clinical Research   1

1   Introduction to R and OpenBUGS   3

1.1   Introduction to R 3
1.2   How to Install R 4
1.3   Packages 4
1.4   How to Install RStudio 6
1.5   OpenBUGS 7

2   Sample Size Determination   13

2.1   Introduction 13
2.2   The Sample Size Formula 14
2.3   Measured Outcomes 15
     2.3.1   Time to event endpoints 15
     2.3.2   Sample size with event-driven trials 16
2.4   Bayesian Sample Size Determination 18
2.5   Study Objective and Sample Size Determination 19
2.6   Bayesian Survival Analysis Sample Size Calculation with R 22
2.7   Illustration 22
2.8   Posterior Error Approach 23
2.9   Different Sample Size Determination Packages in R 23
     2.9.1   BAEssd 23
     2.9.2   BayesianPower 24
     2.9.3   NPHMC 25
     2.9.4   PowerTOST 26
     2.9.5   SampleSize4ClinicalTrials 26
     2.9.6   SSRMST 27
     2.9.7   powerSurvEpi 28
     2.9.8   SampleSizeMeans 28

3 **Study Design-I**   **31**

   3.1   Introduction   31
   3.2   Bayesian in Early Phase Oncology Trial   32
        3.2.1   Rule-based designs   32
               3.2.1.1   3+3 design   33
               3.2.1.2   Pharmacologically guided dose escalation .   33
               3.2.1.3   Accelerated titration designs   34
        3.2.2   Model-based designs for determining the MTD   34
               3.2.2.1   Continual reassessment method (CRM) . .   34
   3.3   Study Design Package Using R   35

4 **Study Design-II**   **39**

   4.1   Introduction   39
   4.2   Methods   41
        4.2.1   Estimating treatment success   41
        4.2.2   Treatment difference testing   42
   4.3   Illustration with Bayesian Using R   43
   4.4   Discussion   46

5 **Optimum Biological Dose Selection**   **47**

   5.1   Introduction   47
   5.2   Illustration with Head and Neck Cancer Data   48
   5.3   Toxicity Profile Testing   48
   5.4   Logistic Response Model   49
   5.5   Dose Selection Algorithm   51
   5.6   Quadratic Logistic Design   52
   5.7   Illustration   53
   5.8   Bayesian Dose Selection Using OpenBUGS   57
   5.9   Discussion   59
   5.10 Dose Finding Package Using R   60
        5.10.1 DoseFinding   60

II **Bayesian in Time-to-Event Data Analysis**   **63**

6 **Survival Analysis**   **65**

   6.1   Introduction   65
        6.1.1   Kaplan-Meier estimator   66
        6.1.2   Nelson-Aalen estimator   67
   6.2   Bayesian in Survival Analysis   68
        6.2.1   Cox's proportional hazards model   68
        6.2.2   Hazard ratio   69
        6.2.3   Partial likelihood function   69

Contents   ix

        6.2.4   Stratified Cox model   70
        6.2.5   Wald-score and likelihood ratio tests   71
        6.2.6   Diagnostics for Cox's PH model   71
        6.2.7   Schoenfeld residuals   72
    6.3   Bayesian Survival Analysis Using R   73
        6.3.1   BayesSurvival   76
        6.3.2   muhaz   76
        6.3.3   Bayesian in Kaplan-meier estimator   76
        6.3.4   Bayesian Cox proportional hazards model   79

7 Competing Risk Data Analysis   87

    7.1   Introduction   87
    7.2   Competing Risk as Bivariate Random Variable   88
    7.3   Cumulative Incidence Rate   89
    7.4   Competing Risk Model Using R   89
    7.5   Cause-Specific Hazard Model   91
    7.6   Bayesian Information Criteria   92
    7.7   Illustration Using R   94

8 Frailty Data Analysis   97

    8.1   Introduction   97
    8.2   Frailty Model   99
    8.3   Motivating Example   99
    8.4   Bayesian in Frailty Survival 104
        8.4.1   Frailty modeling 104
        8.4.2   Frailty on recurrent events 104
        8.4.3   Generalized accelerated failure time (GAFT) frailty
                model 105
        8.4.4   Illustration with leukemia data using R 105

9 Relative Survival Analysis   111

    9.1   Introduction 111
    9.2   Relative Survival Analysis 113
    9.3   Data Methodology 114
    9.4   Illustration with R 115
    9.5   Piecewise Hazard Function 118
    9.6   Piecewise Hazard testing 118
    9.7   Piecewise Hazard Function Analysis 120
    9.8   Different Relative Survival Analysis Package with R   120
        9.8.1   flexrsurv 120
        9.8.2   relsurv 123
        9.8.3   survexp.fr 124
    9.9   Discussion 127

III   Bayesian in Longitudinal Data Analysis   129

10 Longitudinal Data Analysis   131

    10.1   Introduction   131
    10.2   Advantages of Longitudinal Analysis   132
    10.3   Limitation of Longitudinal Analysis   132
    10.4   Mixed Effect Model   132
    10.5   Different R Packages for Longitudinal Data Analysis   133
    10.6   Random-Effect Model with R   134
        10.6.1 bayeslongitudinal   134
    10.7   Illustration with Quality of Life Using OpenBUGS   136
    10.8   Result   140

11 Missing Data Analysis   143

    11.1   Introduction   143
    11.2   Different Types of Missing Data   144
        11.2.1 Missing completely at random (MCAR)   144
        11.2.2 Missing at random (MAR)   144
        11.2.3 Missing not at random (NMAR)   144
    11.3   Different Softwares   145
    11.4   Illustration with Lung Cancer Data   145
    11.5   Different Package for Missing Data with R   146
        11.5.1 BMTAR   146
        11.5.2 NestedCohort   148
    11.6   Conclusion   151

12 Joint Longitudinal and Survival Analysis   153

    12.1   Introduction   153
    12.2   Data Methodology   154
    12.3   The Longitudinal Model   155
    12.4   The Survival Model   155
    12.5   The Joint Model   156
    12.6   Submodels Specification   156
    12.7   Different R Package for Joint Longitudinal Model   165
        12.7.1 joint.Cox   165
        12.7.2 JM   166

13 Covariance Modeling   169

    13.1   Introduction   169
    13.2   Covariance Patterns   170
    13.3   Covariance Patterns Challenges   173
    13.4   Illustration with Protein-Gene Expression Time-Course Data   173

IV Bayesian in Diagnostics Test Statistics   183

14 Bayesian Inference in Mixed-Effect Model   185

14.1 Introduction 185
14.2 Likelihood Function with Doses and Measurement Process . 187
14.3 Linear Mixed-Effects Model 188
14.4 Autoregressive Linear Mixed-Effects Model 189
14.5 Linear Mixed-Effects Model Compatible with Dose Response 189
14.6 Autoregressive Linear Mixed Effects Model Compatible with
      Dose Response 190
14.7 Generating Data 190
14.8 Computation Support 192
14.9 Power Analysis of the Performed Models 194
14.10 Discussion 194

15 Concordance Analysis   197

15.1 Introduction 197
15.2 Computational Methodology 199
15.3 Bayes Factor 202
15.4 Results 203
15.5 Conclusion 206

16 High-Dimensional Data Analysis   209

16.1 Introduction 209
16.2 Heatmap with R 210
16.3 Principal Component Analysis with R 212
16.4 Penalized Partial Log-Likelihood (PLL) 213
16.5 Estimating the Predictive PLL 214
16.6 Integrated Prediction Error Curve (IPEC) 214
16.7 Ridge Estimators in Cox Regression 214
16.8 High-Dimensional Data Analysis Using R 215
16.9 Different Packages with R 222
      16.9.1 BAMA 222
      16.9.2 countgmifs 223
      16.9.3 fastcox 223
      16.9.4 HighDimOut 224
16.10 Discussion 226

Bibliography   227

Index   241

Preface

Over the past decades, computational flexibility has extended the application of the Bayesian approach as a handy method in research practice. The oncology disease complexity and existing challenge to obtain the best therapeutic effect has provided immense opportunity to develop the statistical methodology. Perhaps, the acceptance of the Bayesian approach in oncology research is relatively low. There is a vast scope to extend the analytical approach by Bayesian in oncology research practice. This book intended to make a single source of information on Bayesian statistical methodology for oncology research to cover several dimensions like study design, sample size calculation, time-to-event data analysis, and diagnostics implication. The idea is to overall extending the Bayesian approach in oncology research practice.

This book is structured with four sections to extend Bayesian in oncology research. Study design-related topics proposed to bring in Part I. The importance of statistics in the oncology domain first felt during the setup of the required participant's size for an oncology trial. Chapter 1 gives an introduction about R and OpenBUGS software. It is prepared to understand about basic stuff of R and OpenBUGS.

Now Chapter 2 is explained with sample size determination. The Bayesian counterpart to calculate the sample size determination presented. An inferiority trial overrules the application of a placebo-controlled trial due to the ethical constraints and availability of several molecules in the oncology domain. Chapter 3 illustrated about conventional study design for oncology clinical trials. The alternative approach of traditional design of study shown in Chapter 4. It is not always that high-dose chemotherapy will work as the best therapeutic arm. Oncology is a complex disease. Sometimes low-dose frequently used chemo regime works well to control the disease progression. The low-dose chemotherapy is decided based on the optimum biological dose (OBD). The Bayesian statistical methodology on low-dose chemotherapy selection procedure demonstrated in Chapter 5.

Section II proposed to develop and present a different statistical approach with real data application with time-to-event data analysis. The conventional technique on survival analysis is a frequentist-based approach and method with Kaplan-Meier and Cox proportional hazard models always performed. However, there is minimal literature support about the Bayesian counterpart on Cox proportional hazard modeling. Chapter 6 shows about Bayesian survival analysis. The competing risk, i.e., cancer patient, died due to other causes than cancer is a new issue in oncology data. The decision about the best therapeutic regime in the presence of competing for risk is always challenging. Chapter 7 is presented with Bayesian competing risk analysis to compare two therapeutic schemes. The concept of frailty provides a convenient way of introducing unobserved heterogeneity and associations into models for survival data. Frailty is an unobserved random proportionality factor. It influences the hazard function of an individual or related individual chapter 7 prepared on Bayesian frailty data analysis. Similarly, Chapter 8 prepared about Bayesian relative survival analysis. This work developed with an illustration.

In this chapter, we will show with a Bayesian analysis for right-censored survival suitable for curable cancer site data. Bayesian inference with Markov chain Monte Carlo (MCMC) methods will be established through model selection technique and example with a real dataset. The Section III is about statistical methodology in longitudinal and survival data analysis. Bayesian inferences for longitudinal data analysis in oncology research is evitable. It is attractive due to the ability to consider prior information for statistical growth curve modeling. Chapter 10 focused on longitudinal data analysis. The mixed-effect model illustrated with R. The Bayesian inference on missing longitudinal data illustrated in Chapter 11. Similarly, the Bayesian approach is suitable to handle Joint longitudinal and survival data. It helps to consider the dependence between two types of responses obtained by two different methods. In Chapter 12, the joint longitudinal and survival analysis presented. Different prior assumptions and covariance matrix presented with posterior inference. The work performed with OpenBUGS software. Chapter 13 has presented with different covariance structures observed by longitudinal measurements. The Bayesian counterpart illustrated different covariance structures.

The final section-IV is detailed on diagnosis test statistics with available statistical methodology. The author illustrated the Bayesian method to provide inference on different inter and intra-rater agreement analyzes. Chapter 14 is present about mixed effect modeling. It is dedicated to select the specific dose in oncology. Chapter 15 is dedicated to concordance analysis by the Bayesian approach. The CCC is a useful tool in agreement analysis. The importance of high-dimensional data in oncology research will be explored. The Bayesian approach in high-dimensional data is in Chapter 16. The R and OpenBUGS codes illustrated.

Author

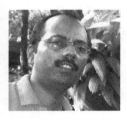Atanu Bhattacharjee is an Assistant Professor at the Section of Biostatistics, Centre for Cancer Epidemiology, Tata Memorial Centre, India. He previously taught Biostatistics at the Malabar Cancer Centre, Kerala, India. He completed his PhD at Gauhati University, Assam, on Bayesian Statistical Inference. He is an elected member of the International Biometric Society (Indian Region). He served as Associate Editor of BMC Medical Research Methodology. He has published over 200 research articles in various peer-reviewed journals.

Part I

Bayesian in Clinical Research

Chapter 1

Introduction to R and OpenBUGS

Abstract

This chapter starts with the history of R software development. Steps to install R are discussed. It provides about the installation of different packages in R.Graphical representation by R will help many users to get interested in a graphical illustration.Steps to install R studio. Description of OpenBUGS software and illustration to perform Markov Chain Monte Carlo in OpenBUGS. Introduction about Bayesian using Gibbs sampling accessible. Different types of Markov chain Monte Carlo (MCMC) approaches are outlined. OpenBUGS model explanation, trace plot generation, data loading and posterior estimates generation are described. The real-world examples are used to illustrate the methods presented. It should provide some familiarity about the R process and essentially environment on what actually works. R software works as the integration of data calculation, graphical procedure, and data manipulation. Command to work with R is presented. This chapter did not explain about statistics in R. The aim is to provide R and OpenBUGS environment. It is preferred to show the environment to work with the classical and modern statistical test to implement. Illustrations are presented by the workstations with windows system. It will guide the users about the available facility.

1.1 Introduction to R

R is a programming language developed by Ross Ihaka and Robert Gentleman in 1993. It is a free software for graphics and statistical computing. The source code of R is prepared primarily in Fortran, R, and C. Although R works are command-driven software, there are other graphical user interfaces like RStudio. R is named partly after the first names of the first two R authors and partly as a play on the name of S [1].

There are several dedicated R packages available in R for specific statistical methods. However, linear modeling, nonlinear modeling, time-series analysis, clustering, and other analysis can be performed in R itself. No special packages are required to install. The R community is noted for its active contributions in terms of packages. R users typically access the command-line interpreted. For example, if the user types 4+4 at the command prompt and press enter, the computer replies with 8, as shown below.

```
>4+4
>8
```

RStudio is an integrated development environment (IDE) for R. It is basically a nice front-end for R, giving you a console, a scripting window, a graphics window, and an R workspace, among other options.

1.2   How to Install R

1. Download R from: http://cran.us.r-project.org/ (click on "Download R for Windows" > "base"> "Download R 3.6.2 for Windows").
2. Install R. Leave all default settings in the installation options.

1.3   Packages

The datasets and functions available in R are stored in packages. A specific package is needed to install before its contents available. The packages available can be obtained as

```
> library()
```

To see which packages are currently loaded, use

```
> search()
```

The standard (or base) packages are defined as part of the R source code. This contains the essential functions that allow R to work. Datasets and standard statistical and graphical functions are available. Data can be generated from the normal distribution by 'rnorm' as

```
#Generate Data Distribution

x <- rnorm(50)
y <- rnorm(x)
plot(x, y)
```

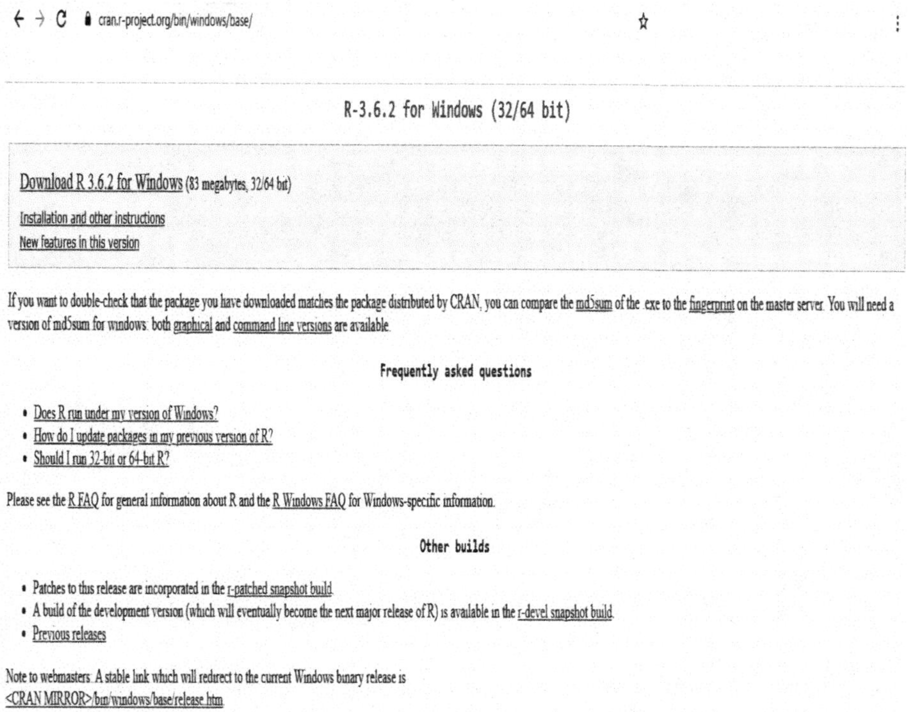

← → C 🔒 cran.r-project.org/bin/windows/base/ ☆ ⋮

R-3.6.2 for Windows (32/64 bit)

<u>Download R 3.6.2 for Windows</u> (83 megabytes, 32/64 bit)

<u>Installation and other instructions</u>
<u>New features in this version</u>

If you want to double-check that the package you have downloaded matches the package distributed by CRAN, you can compare the <u>md5sum</u> of the exe to the <u>fingerprint</u> on the master server. You will need a version of md5sum for windows: both <u>graphical</u> and <u>command line versions</u> are available.

Frequently asked questions

* <u>Does R run under my version of Windows?</u>
* <u>How do I update packages in my previous version of R?</u>
* <u>Should I run 32-bit or 64-bit R?</u>

Please see the <u>R FAQ</u> for general information about R and the <u>R Windows FAQ</u> for Windows-specific information.

Other builds

* Patches to this release are incorporated in the <u>r-patched snapshot build</u>.
* A build of the development version (which will eventually become the next major release of R) is available in the <u>r-devel snapshot build</u>.
* <u>Previous releases</u>

Note to webmasters: A stable link which will redirect to the current Windows binary release is
<CRAN MIRROR>/bin/windows/base/release.htm

FIGURE 1.1: How to download R software.

```
#Generate Line Plot with R

chemotreated <- c(105,112,110,90,109,115)
radiothrapytreated <- c(120,127,132,125,127,118)
grange <- range(0,chemotreated,radiothrapytreated)
plot(chemotreated, type="o", col="blue", ylim=grange,
axes=FALSE, ann=FALSE)
axis(1, at=1:5, lab=c("Mon","Tue","Wed","Thu","Fri"))
axis(2, las=1, at=4*0:grange[2])
box()
lines(radiothrapytreated, type="o", pch=22, lty=2, col="red")
title(main="Chemo and Radiation Given Patients", col.main="red",
font.main=4)
title(xlab="Days", col.lab=rgb(0,0.5,0))
title(ylab="Total Treated Patients", col.lab=rgb(0,0.5,0))
legend(1,50, c("Chemo","Radiation"), cex=0.8,
col=c("blue","red"), pch=21:22, lty=1:2);
```

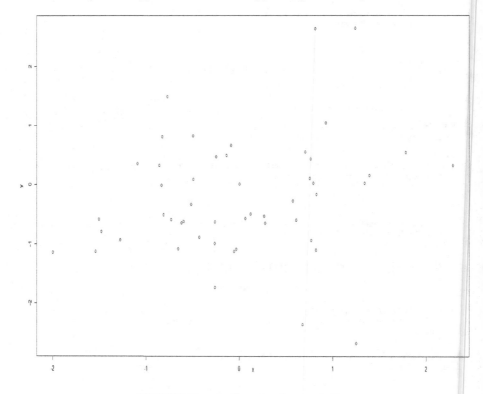

FIGURE 1.2: Simple plot with R.

Now the Plot function is useful. A graphics window will appear automatically. There are thousands of functions available in R. This function can be obtained from the Comprehensive R Archive Network (CRAN): https://cran.r-project.org.

1.4   How to Install RStudio

1. Download RStudio from: http://rstudio.org/download/desktop and install it. Leave all default settings in the installation options.
2. Open RStudio.
3. Go to the "Packages" tab and click on "Install Packages". The first time it will prompt to choose a CRAN mirror.
4. R will download all necessary files from the server to select here. Choose the location closest to your geographical location.
5. Install packages in Windows.

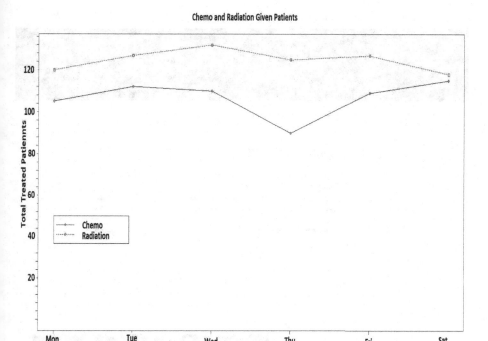

FIGURE 1.3: Line plot with R.

1.5 OpenBUGS

BUGS is an open source statistical software package used for Bayesian inference using Gibbs sampling. The statistical model is specified by merely stating the relationship between covariates and outcome variables. The MCMC technique is used for analyzing the specified model. It can be downloaded from: http://www.openbugs.net/w/Downloads. A setup program for Open-BUGS on Windows computers is available. The latest version is available as version 3.2.2. The manual is also available over there.

It is better to have knowledge of MCMC methods to work with Open-BUGS. There are three different families of MCMC algorithms like Gibbs, Metropolis-Hastings, and slice sampling to work with OpenBUGS. Primarily, Gibbs sampling algorithm works to sample from the conditional distribution of each node given for all the others in the graph. It works as a particular case of Metropolis-Hastings algorithm.

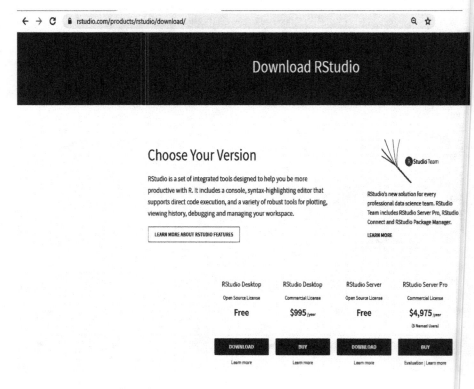

FIGURE 1.4: Selection of free RStudio version.

The OpenBUGS is used to define the concise expression of the model, by the 'twiddles' symbol $\sim$. This symbol is used to define the stochastic (probabilistic) relationships. Thereafter, the left arrow ' $<$ ' followed by '-' is used to define the relationship between outcome and covariates. The model is defined as:

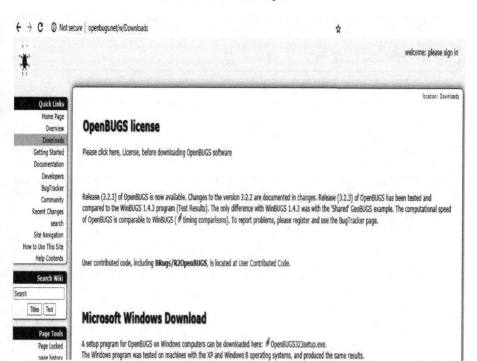

FIGURE 1.5: How to install OpenBUGS.

```
#Define OpenBUGS Model

model
{
for (i in 1 : Dogs) {
xa[i, 1] <- 0; xs[i, 1] <- 0 p[i, 1] <- 0
for (j in 2 : Trials) {
xa[i, j] <- sum(Y[i, 1 : j - 1])
xs[i, j] <- j - 1 - xa[i, j]
log(p[i, j]) <- alpha × xa[i, j] + beta × xs[i, j]
y[i, j] <- 1 - Y[i, j]
y[i, j] ~ dbern(p[i, j])
}
}
alpha ~ dnorm(0, 0.00001)I(, -0.00001)
beta ~ dnorm(0, 0.00001)I(, -0.00001)
A <- exp(alpha)
B <- exp(beta)
}
```

#Define Initial Data

list(alpha = -1, beta = -1)

Now at step 1, we select the model.

Now at step 2, we will check the model description and look it runs appropriately or not.

At the next step, we should load the data.

Now at step 4, we need to select the number of chains (i.e., sets of samples to simulate). The default is 1, but we will use two chains for this tutorial.

#Define Data

list(Dogs = 30, Trials = 25, Y = structure(.Data = c(0, 0, 1, 0, 1, 0, 1, 1, 1, 1, 1, 1, 1, 1, 1, 1, 1, 1, 1, 1, 1, 1, 1, 0, 0, 0, 0, 0, 0, 0, 1, 0, 0, 0, 0, 0, 0, 1, 1, 1, 1, 1, 1, 1, 1, 1, 1, 0, 0, 0, 0, 0, 1, 1, 0, 1, 1, 0, 0, 1, 1, 0, 1, 0, 1, 1, 1, 1, 1, 1, 1, 0, 1, 1, 0, 0, 1, 1, 1, 1, 0, 1, 0, 1, 0, 1, 1, 1, 1, 1, 1, 1, 1, 1, 0, 0, 0, 0, 0, 0, 0, 1, 1, 1, 1, 1, 1, 1, 1, 1, 1, 1, 1, 1, 1, 1, 0, 0, 0, 0, 0, 0, 1, 1, 1, 1, 0, 0, 1, 0, 1, 1, 1, 1, 1, 1, 1, 1, 1, 1, 1, 0, 0, 0, 0, 0, 1, 0, 0, 0, 0, 0, 0, 1, 1, 1, 1, 1, 1, 1, 1, 1, 1, 1, 1, 1, 1, 1, 0, 0, 0, 1, 0, 0, 0, 1, 1, 0, 0, 1, 1, 1, 1, 1, 1, 1, 1, 1, 1, 1, 1, 1, 1, 0, 0, 0, 0, 0, 1, 0, 1, 0, 1, 0, 0, 0, 1, 1, 1, 1, 1, 0, 1, 1, 0, 0, 0, 0, 0, 0, 1, 0, 0, 1, 1, 0, 1, 0, 1, 1, 1, 1, 1, 1, 1, 1, 1, 1, 1, 1, 0, 0, 0, 0, 0, 0, 0, 0, 0, 0, 1, 1, 1, 1, 1, 1, 1, 1, 1, 1, 1, 1, 1, 1, 1, 1, 0, 0, 0, 0, 0, 1, 1, 1, 1, 1, 0, 0, 1, 1, 1, 1, 1, 1, 1, 1, 1, 1, 1, 1, 1, 1, 0, 0, 0, 1, 1, 0, 1, 0, 0, 1, 1, 1, 1, 1, 1, 1, 1, 1, 1, 0, 0, 0, 0, 1, 0, 1, 1, 0, 1, 0, 1, 1, 1, 1, 1, 1, 1, 1, 1, 1, 1, 1, 1, 1, 0, 0, 0, 1, 0, 1, 1, 0, 1, 1, 0, 1, 1, 1, 1, 1, 1, 1, 1, 1, 1, 1, 1, 1, 1, 1, 1, 0, 0, 0, 0, 0, 0, 0, 1, 1, 1, 1, 1, 1, 1, 1, 1, 1, 1, 1, 1, 1, 1, 1, 1, 0, 1, 0, 1, 0, 0, 0, 1, 0, 1, 1, 1, 0, 1, 1, 1, 1, 1, 1, 1, 1, 1, 1, 1, 1, 1, 1, 0, 0, 0, 1, 0, 1, 0, 1, 1, 1, 1, 1, 0, 1, 1, 1, 1, 1, 1, 1, 1, 1, 1, 0, 1, 0, 0, 0, 0, 0, 1, 0, 0, 0, 1, 1, 1, 1, 1, 1, 1, 1, 1, 1, 1, 1, 0, 0, 0, 0, 1, 1, 0, 1, 0, 1, 1, 0, 1, 0, 1, 0, 1, 1, 1, 1, 1, 1, 1, 1, 1, 1, 1, 1, 0, 0, 0, 1, 1, 1, 1, 1, 1, 1, 1, 1, 1, 0, 0, 1, 0, 1, 0, 1, 1, 1, 1, 1, 1, 1, 1, 1, 1, 0, 0, 0, 1, 0, 1, 0, 1, 1, 1, 1, 1, 1, 1, 1, 1, 1, 1, 0, 0, 0, 1, 1, 1, 1, 1, 0, 1, 1, 1, 1, 1, 1, 1, 1, 1, 0, 0, 1, 0, 1, 0, 1, 1, 1, 1, 1, 1, 1, 0, 0, 0, 0, 0, 0, 0, 1, 1, 1, 1, 1, 1, 1, 1, 1, 1, 1, 1, 1, 1, 1, 1, 0, 0, 0, 0, 0, 0, 0, 0, 1, 1, 1, 0, 1, 0, 0, 0, 1, 1, 0, 1, 1, 1, 1, 1, 0, 0, 0, 0, 0, 1, 1, 0, 1, 1, 1, 0, 1, 0, 1, 1, 1, 1, 1, 1, 1, 1, 1, 1, 1, 0, 0, 1, 0, 1, 1, 1, 0, 1, 1, 0, 1, 1, 1, 1, 1, 1, 1, 1, 1, 1, 1, 1, 1, 1, 1, 0, 0, 0, 0, 1, 0, 1, 1, 1, 1, 1, 1, 1, 1, 1, 1, 1, 1, 1, 1, 1, 1, 1, 1, 0, 0, 0, 1, 0, 1, 0, 1, 1, 1, 0, 1, 1, 1, 1, 1, 1, 1, 1, 1, 1, 1, 1, 1, 1, 0, 0, 0, 0, 0, 1, 1, 0, 0, 1, 1, 0, 1, 0, 1, 0, 1, 0, 1, 1, 1, 1, 1, 1, 1, 0, 0, 0, 0, 0, 1, 1, 1, 1, 1, 1, 0, 1, 0, 1, 1, 1, 1, 1, 1, 1, 1, 1, 1, 1, 1, 1), .Dim = c(30, 25)))

#Results					
mean	sd	MC error	val2.5pc	median	val97.5pc
alpha	0.24	0.027	0.00	− 0.29	− 0.24
beta	− 0.07	0.018	0.00	− 0.10	− 0.07

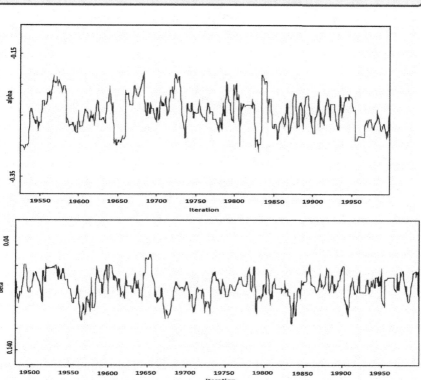

FIGURE 1.6: Trace plot example in OpenBUGS.

Chapter 2

Sample Size Determination

Abstract

The sample size for a clinical trial jointly works with study design. A different issue like a number of sites, number of treatments also considered for sample size determination. The appropriate response plays an essential role in sample size calculation. Computing large sample size always wastes of time, money and unnecessarily put patients into a risk. Similarly, sample size too small always makes a less powerful statement. Thus, it is essential to compute sample size wisely to decide minimal clinically meaningful effect size with pre-specified type I error and power. It is not possible to plan a clinical trial unless we know the required sample size. However, there is a different strategy to perform any oncology trial. The study design and study hypothesis play a combined role to determine the sample size. There are some great sample size and power calculation software packages available. We presented this chapter with some R sample size calculation packages. However, there are undoubtedly other packages that you might consider. The R packages are illustrated toward implementing Bayesian for sample size calculation. Theoretical explanation about Bayesian Sample size determination is discussed. Different R packages are used to solve the problem and all of the problems that encountered do a better job the other on certain types of scenario.

2.1   Introduction

How many subjects do we need? How long will the study take to complete? In survival analysis, we need to specify information regarding the censoring mechanism and the particular survival distributions in the null and alternative hypotheses.

First, one needs either to specify what parametric survival model to use, or that the test will be semi-parametric, e.g., the log-rank test. It requires to determining the number of deaths (or events) required to meet the power and other design specifications.

Second, one must also provide an estimate of the number of patients that need to entered into the trial to produce the required number of deaths. We shall assume that the patients enter a trial over a certain accrual period of length a, and then followed for an additional period f known as the follow-up time. Patients still alive at the end of follow-up are censored. Sample size calculations are an essential part of study design Consider sample size requirements early.

A well-designed trial is large enough to detect clinically important differences between groups with high probability.

To perform sample size calculations, we need well-defined study endpoints, hypotheses, and statistical tests. Study hypotheses decided on a clearly defined endpoint and period of study.

In most RCTs, known as superiority trials, the study hypothesis presented as a null hypothesis of no difference in the distribution of the primary endpoint between study groups. We have an alternative hypothesis in mind, for example: H_A. The frequency of events at 30 days will differ in the two treatment groups.

In superiority trials, we test the null hypothesis against a two-sided alternative. When we test the null hypothesis, there are two possible states of nature and two decisions: We will perform a test that has a small probability of a Type 1 error, usually 0.05. The power of the study is the probability that we will reject the null hypothesis when the alternative hypothesis is true. We want this probability to be large, typically at least 0.8.

2.2 The Sample Size Formula

$$n = \frac{2\bar{p} * (1 - \bar{p})(Z_{\alpha/2} + Z_\beta)^2}{\Delta^2} \tag{2.1}$$

$Z_{\alpha/2}$ and Z_β are the critical values of the normal distribution, $\bar{p}$ is the average of the event rates under the alternative hypothesis, and Δ is the true difference under H_A.

For example, $\alpha = 0.05, \beta = 0.20, 2n = 1,903$ or n $= 806$.

2.3 Measured Outcomes

If we are testing the equality of two treatments (T and C), and the endpoint is a measurement, the null hypothesis is typically expressed in terms of the difference in means

$$-\text{True Means} : \mu_T = \mu_C \qquad (2.2)$$

$$-\text{Difference} : \Delta = \mu_T - \mu_C \qquad (2.3)$$

$$-H_0 : \Delta = 0, H_\alpha : \Delta > 0 \text{ or} \Delta < 0 \qquad (2.4)$$

2.3.1 Time to event endpoints

In many clinical trials, the primary endpoint is the time to an event, e.g., death or disease progression.
In that circumstance, the analyst will employ methods specific to the analysis of "survival data".
We discuss those methods briefly here, but in greater detail later in the course.
Estimate the survival distribution in each treatment group and use nonparametric methods to compare them.
The most common test is known as the log-rank test.
Modern methods accommodate variable entry times and periods of follow-up.
The standard nonparametric test for comparing two distributions is the log-rank test.
Interestingly, sample size formulas for the log-rank test are closely related to those that apply when the times-to-event follow an exponential distribution.
With exponential survival distributions, the null hypothesis is $H_0 : \lambda_T = \lambda_C$

A simple formula for the sample size, assuming all subjects are followed to the event, is

$$n = 2(Z_{\alpha/2} + Z_\beta)^2/[\ln(\lambda_C/\lambda_T)]^2 \qquad (2.5)$$

where the values of λ_C and λ_T are given by H_A. If the subjects are recruited over some time, and the study ends when some items have not had the event, sample size calculations are more complex
Lachin formula [2]

$$n = (Z_{\alpha/2} + Z_\beta)[\phi(\lambda_T) + \phi(\lambda_C)]/(\lambda_T - \lambda_C)^2 \qquad (2.6)$$

The sample size depends on the recruitment and follow-up schedules.

2.3.2   Sample size with event-driven trials

For the logrank test, the power of the study depends on the number of events observed. This has led to the concept of the event-driven trial. Schoenfeld showed that, if the logrank test will be used to compare two time-to-event distributions, the number of events required to achieve power of $1 - \beta$ is

$$n = 4(z_{\alpha/2} + z_\beta)^2/[\ln(\lambda_C/\lambda_T)]^2 \tag{2.7}$$

```
#Sample Size Calculation with R

library("gsDesign")
ss <- nSurvival(lambda1=.2, lambda2=.1, eta = .1,
Ts = 2, Tr = .5,sided=1, alpha=.025)
ss
```

```
# R Output

Fixed design, two-arm trial with time-to-event
outcome (Lachin and Foulkes, 1986).
Study duration (fixed):        Ts=2
Accrual duration (fixed):      Tr=0.5
Uniform accrual:           entry="unif"
Control median:        log(2)/lambda1=3.5
Experimental median: log(2)/lambda2=6.9
Censoring median:         log(2)/eta=6.9
Control failure rate:      lambda1=0.2
Experimental failure rate:  lambda2=0.1
Censoring rate:            eta=0.1
Power:               100*(1-beta)=90%
Type I error (1-sided):   100*alpha=2.5%
Equal randomization:        ratio=1
Sample size based on hazard ratio=0.5 (type="rr")
Sample size (computed):        n=430
Events required (computed): nEvents=91
```

```
# Sample Size Calculation with R

library("gsDesign")
x<-gsDesign(k = 5, test.type = 2, n.fix=ss$nEvents,
nFixSurv=ss$n,delta1=log(ss$lambda2/ss$lambda1))

x
```

```
#R Output
```

```
Group sequential design sample size for time-to-event outcome
with sample size 440. The analysis plan below shows events
at each analysis.
Symmetric two-sided group sequential design with
90 % power and 2.5 % Type I Error.
Spending computations assume trial stops
if a bound is crossed.
  Analysis N   Z   Nominal p  Spend
         1 19 3.25   0.0006 0.0006
         2 37 2.99   0.0014 0.0013
         3 56 2.69   0.0036 0.0028
         4 74 2.37   0.0088 0.0063
         5 93 2.03   0.0214 0.0140
     Total                   0.0250
++ alpha spending:
 Hwang-Shih-DeCani spending function with gamma = -4.
Boundary crossing probabilities and expected sample size
assume any cross stops the trial
Upper boundary (power or Type I Error)
         Analysis
   Theta     1      2      3      4      5 Total E{N}
  0.0000 0.0006 0.0013 0.0028 0.0063 0.0140 0.025 91.5
  0.3415 0.0370 0.1512 0.2647 0.2699 0.1771 0.900 66.4
Lower boundary (futility or Type II Error)
         Analysis
   Theta     1      2      3      4      5 Total
  0.0000 6e-04 0.0013 0.0028 0.0063 0.014 0.025
  0.3415 0e+00 0.0000 0.0000 0.0000 0.000 0.000
```

```
#Sample Size Calculation for the Comparison of Survival Curves Com-
parison
```

```
library("powerSurvEpi")
ssizeCT.default(power = 0.8,k = 1,pE=0.3707,
pC = 0.4890,RR = 0.7,alpha = 0.05)
```

2.4   Bayesian Sample Size Determination

It is not possible to plan a clinical trial unless we know the required sample size. However, there is a different strategy to perform any oncology trial. The study design and study hypothesis play a combined role to determine the sample size. Conventionally approach is to consideration of comparison to the existing arm. Now the interpretation can be separated as a null and alternative hypothesis. Under the null hypothesis, it is assumed that the experimental and exsisting arms similar. The outcome is survival. Now the survival outcome can be formulated as an event/event-free at a specific time point. Now it can be death or relapse. Determination of event size is required to perform any oncology clinical trial. It may be an event number of sample size. Suppose we have two types of treatment for head and neck cancer defined as Arm A and Arm B. The prior information about death probability those are treated with Arm-A is 40% after the end of 3 -years. Similarly, it is 50% after three years for those who are treated with Arm-B. Now the null hypothesis is formulated as $H_0 : P_A = P_B$. The alternative hypothesis can be formulated as $H_1 : P_A \neq P_B$. The level of significance is defined as α, and type-II error is defined as β. The level of importance can be defined as a type-I error. The task is about balancing the type-I and type-II error to get the optimum sample size. Suppose the sample size for trial 1 and 2 are calculated as n_1 and n_2. Both trials are designed for the same treatment effect. Now the success of those trials is defined as π_1 and π_1 respectively. The parameter π_1 and π_2 are measured as x_1/n_1 and x_2/n_2 respectively. The number of patients alive after the end of 3 years for both the trial are x_1 and x_2 respectively. Now the posterior distribution is presented as

$$f(\pi_1, \pi_2 | x_1, x_2, n_1, n_2) = k f(\pi_1, \pi_2) \prod_{i=1}^{2} \pi_i^{x_i} (1 - \pi_i)^{n_i - x_i} \qquad (2.8)$$

The normalizing constant is prepared as k. The posterior dsitribution is dependent on the prior distribution. Now π_1 and π_2 can calculated from beta distributions with paramters (c_1, d_1) and (c_2, d_2), respectively. The equation can be formulated as

$$f(\pi_1, \pi_2 | x_1, x_2, n_1, n_2) = k \prod_{i=1}^{2} \pi_i^{x_i + c_i - 1} (1 - \pi_i)^{n_i - x_i + d_i - 1} \qquad (2.9)$$

Now

$$k = [B(x_1 + c_1, n_1 - x_1 + d_1) B(x_2 + c_2, n_2 - x_2 + d_2)]^{-1} \qquad (2.10)$$

and $B(.,.)$ represents the beta function. The term (x_1, x_2) can be formulated as

$$p(x_1, x_2) = \prod_{i=1}^{2} \frac{\binom{n_i}{x_i} B(x_i + c_i, n_i - x_i + d_i)}{B(c_i, d_i)} \tag{2.11}$$

The simplified form of joint posterior distribution can be formulated as

$$f(\pi_1, \theta | x_1, x_2, n_1, n_2) = k\pi_1^{x_1 + x_1 - 1}(1 - \pi_1)^{n_1 - x_1 + d_1 - 1}$$
$$(\pi_1 - \theta)^{x_2 + c_2 - 1}(1 - \pi_1 + \theta)^{n_2 - x_2 + d_2 - 1} \tag{2.12}$$

which is non-zero over the region in the plane bounded by the lines $\pi_1 = 0, \pi_1 = 1, \pi_1 = \theta$ and $\pi_1 = \theta + 1$. The marginal posterior distribution of θ can be formulated as

$$f(\theta | x_1, x_2, n_1, n_2) = \int_{\max(0,\theta)}^{\min(\theta+1,1)} f(\pi_1, \theta | x_1, x_2, n_1, n_2) d\pi_1 \tag{2.13}$$

2.5 Study Objective and Sample Size Determination

The sample size for a clinical trial jointly works with study design. A different issue like a number of sites, number of treatment also considered for sample size determination. The appropriate response plays an essential role in sample size calculation. Computing large sample size always wastes of time, money and unnecessarily put patients into a risk. Similarly, sample size too small always makes a less powerful statement Thus, it is essential to compute sample size wisely to decide minimal clinically meaningful effect size with prespecified type I error and power. Hypothesis testing and statistical test are two crucial part in sample size calculation. Initially, the null and alternative hypothesis need to be specified. Therefore proper statistical analysis needs to be determined.Sample size can be specified with type-I error and power of $1 - \beta$, effect size, and other design related parameter. Suppose that the null hypothesis with the probability of survival after 3/5 years of treatment initiation is specified as p_1 and p_2 for arm A and arm B. The null hypothesis is defined as

$$H_0 : p_1 \leq p_2 \quad \text{vs} \quad H_1 : p_1 > p_2 \tag{2.14}$$

The study is powered with alternative hypothesis as $p = p_1(< p_2)$. Now, given the type I error α and power of $1 - \beta$ under the alternative $H_1 : p = p_1$. The effect size is $\omega = p_2 - p_1 > 0$. The sample size is calculated based on the following assumptions. The statistics U under the H_0 is asymptotically normal distributed with mean p_1 and variance σ_0^2/n.

Let $\hat{\sigma}^2$ is a consistent estimator of σ_0^2. The null hypothesis is

$$Z = \frac{\sqrt{n}(U - \mu_0)}{\hat{\sigma}} \to N(0,1) \tag{2.15}$$

Here Z converges to normal distribution with mean zero and variance 1.

$$\Phi(x) = \int_{-\infty}^{x} \frac{1}{\sqrt{2\pi}} exp^{-\frac{u^2}{2}} du \tag{2.16}$$

Under the one-sided test, we reject the H_0 if $Z > z_{1-\alpha}$ Now, $z_{1-\alpha} = 1 - \alpha$ percentile of the standard normal distribution and $z_{1-\alpha} = \Phi^{-1}(1-\alpha)$. Under the alternative $p_1 = p_2, \sigma^2$ converges to σ^2. It is assumed that Z is asymptotically normal distributed with mean $\sqrt{n}\omega/\sigma$ and unit variance. The power $1 - \beta$ is defined as an alternative $p_0 = p_2$. It present with the equations:

$$1 - \beta = P(Z > z_{1-\alpha}|H_1) = P(\frac{\sqrt{n}(U - \mu_0)}{\hat{\sigma}} > z_{1-\alpha}|H_1) \tag{2.17}$$

$$1 - \beta = P(Z > z_{1-\alpha}|H_1) = P(\frac{\sqrt{n}(U - \mu_0)}{\hat{\sigma}} > z_{1-\alpha} - \frac{\sqrt{n}\omega}{\sigma}|H_1) \tag{2.18}$$

$$1 - \beta = P(Z > z_{1-\alpha}|H_1) \simeq \Phi(-z_{1-\alpha} + \frac{\sqrt{n}\omega}{\sigma}) \tag{2.19}$$

$(z_{1-\alpha} + z_{1-\beta}) = \sqrt{n}\omega$
Finally, the sample size is obtained with n by

$$n = \frac{(z_{1-\alpha} + z_{1-\beta})^2\sigma^2}{\omega^2} \tag{2.20}$$

#Average Coverage Criterion (ACC)

The θ pararmeter is used to make different two binomical parameters, it can be specified by minimizing n

$$\sum_{x_1=0}^{n} \sum_{x_2=0}^{n} Pr\{\theta \in (a(x_1, x_2), a(x_1, x_2) + l)\}p(x_1, x_2) \geq 1 - \alpha \tag{2.21}$$

where

$$\sum_{x_1=0}^{n} \sum_{x_2=0}^{n} Pr\{\theta \in (a(x_1, x_2), a(x_1, x_2)+l)\} = \int_{a(x_1,x_2)}^{a(x_1,x_2+l)} f(\theta|x_1, x_2, n)d\theta \tag{2.22}$$

The lower limit of the Highest Posterior Density (HPD) is defined through x_1, x_2. The term probability $1 - \alpha$ varies with x with HPD interval l. It helps to define the sample with minimum size n by

$$\int_{X} \{\int_{a(x,n)}^{a(x,n)+1} f(\theta|x)d\theta\}f(x)dx \geq 1 - \alpha \tag{2.23}$$

#Average Length Criterion (ALC)

The minimum sample size n can be obtained by

$$\sum_{x_1=0}^{n}\sum_{x_2=0}^{n} l^{'}(x_1,x_2)p(x_1,x_2) \leq l \tag{2.24}$$

The HPD is obtained from (x_1,x_2) by solving

$$\int_{a(x_1,x_2)}^{a(x_1,x_2)+l^{'}(x_1,x_2)} f(\theta|x_1,x_2,n) = 1-\alpha \tag{2.25}$$

where $a(x_1,x_2)$ and $a(x_1,x_2)+l^{'}(x_1,x_2)$ are used to cover the HPD interval. In this case the coverage probability is fixed and allows to vary the HPD interval. Length is defined as

$$\int_{a(x,n)}^{a(x,n)+l^{'}(x,n)} f(\theta|x)d\theta = 1-\alpha \tag{2.26}$$

while the sample size is defined as n with minimum integer by

$$\int_X l^{'}(x,n)f(x)dx \leq l \tag{2.27}$$

It is obvious to obtain different sample size through ACC and ALC.

#Worst Outcome Criterion (WOC)

If we fixed the interval with length l and defined the coverage probability with $1-\alpha$ then the minimum sample size n can be defined as

$$\int_{a(x_1^*,x_2^*)}^{a(x_1^*,x_2^*)+l} f(\theta|x_1^*,x_2^*,n)d\theta \geq (1-\alpha) \tag{2.28}$$

The optimum sample size not possible to obtain by ACC and ALC. The conservative approach to maximize the length of l and reduce the minimum coverage probability of $(1-\alpha)$ in connection to the data. The optimum sample size is obtained by

$$\inf_{x\in X}\{\int_{a(x,n)}^{a(x,n)+l} f(\theta|x)d\theta\} \geq 1-\alpha \tag{2.29}$$

It helps to avoid unnecessarily selecting large sample size for clinical trial.

2.6   Bayesian Survival Analysis Sample Size Calculation with R

```
>library("SampleSizeProportions")
```

```
library("SampleSizeProportions")
propdiff.acc(len=0.05, c1=3, d1=2, c2=2, d2=3)
[1] 2483 2483
```

In the above equation the length is defined as the posterior credible interval for the two proportions difference. Now c_1, c_2 are the first priors parameter with Beta density for the first and second population. Similarly d_1, d_2 are the second priors parameter with Beta density for the first and second population. Level of significant is defined as 0.95. Now the calculated sample size for both the groups are (n_1, n_2).

```
propdiff.alc(len=0.05, c1=3, d1=2, c2=3, d2=2)
[1] 2430 2430
```

```
propdiff.mblacc(len=0.05, c1=3, d1=2, c2=2, d2=3)
[1] 2478 2478
```

```
propdiff.mblmodwoc(len=0.05,    c1=3,    d1=2,    c2=2,    d2=3,
worst.level=0.95)
[1] 3070 3070
```

2.7   Illustration

Let there are two experimental arms named as Arm A and Arm B respectively. Arm A is exsisting arm and we want to compare the therapeutic effect of Arm B with reference to Arm A. Now the null hypothesis is required to formulate. The null hypothesis should be linked with sucess of Arm A is similar with Arm B. The success of Arm A is defined as probability of survival of the patients at the end of 3 years is 38%. Similarly, for Arm B it is assumed as 61%. The prior parameters assumption for beta density on Arm A is defined as

3 and 2. Similarly, for Arm B is assumed as 2 and 3. The parameteric assumption with 3 and 2 provides median value as 0.61. Similarly, for arm B as 0.38. There after we fixed the level of significance with 95%. The calculated sample size obtained with ACC for both the arms are 2483. Similarly, we can run the same parameteric assumption with function propdiff.alc,propdiff.mblacc and propdiff.mblmodwoc respectively.

2.8   Posterior Error Approach

The minimum sample size can be obtained by manipulation type-I and type-II error through the frequentist approach. Similarly, the posterior error rate stands to obtain a desirable sample size. The minimum sample size can be obtained so that the posterior error rate can be controlled.It is important to explore the posterior error rate and the relationship with the traditional type I and type II error rate. The posterior error rate is considered as a check and balance of Bayesian sample size calculation.

2.9   Different Sample Size Determination Packages in R

2.9.1   BAEssd

The Bayesian average error approach applicable to estimate the sample size. The function available in BAEssd package named as "norm1KV.2sided" is useful to

```
#BAEssd Package

library("BAEssd")
f1 <- norm1KV.2sided(sigma=5,theta0=0,prob=0.5,mu=2,tau=.1)
ss1 <- ssd.norm1KV.2sided(alpha=0.25,w=0.5,minn=2,maxn=200)
ss1
```

```
#Outcome on BAEssd Package

Sample Size: 34
Total Average Error: 0.2451311
Acceptable sample size determined!
plot(ss1)
plot(ss1,y="AE1",alpha.line=FALSE) abline(h=0.05,lty=2)
```

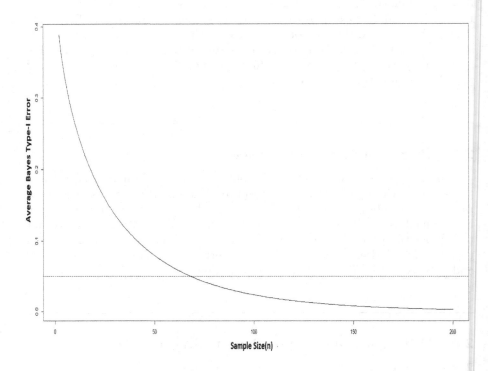

FIGURE 2.1: Type-I error plot on sample size.

2.9.2　BayesianPower

This package is useful to compute the sample size and power for comparing inequality constrained hypotheses. The example of calculating the sample size by "bayes_sampsize" function is in the following text.

```
#Calculating Sample Size by BayesianPower Package

h1 <- matrix(c(1,-1), nrow= 1, byrow= TRUE)
h2 <- 'c'
m1 <- c(.3, 0)
m2 <- c(0, .2)
bayes_sampsize(h1, h2, m1, m2, sd1 = 1, sd2 = 1, scale = 1000,
type = "de" cutoff = .125, nsamp =100, datasets =100,
minss =30, maxss =60)
```

#Inputs Required for BayesianPower Package

n A number. The sample size.
h1 A constraint matrix defining H_1.
h2 A constraint matrix defining H_2.
m1 A vector of expected population means under H_1.
m2 A vector of expected populations means under H_2 .m2 must be of same length as m1.
sd1 A vector of standard deviations under H_1. Must be a single number (equal).
standard deviation under all populations), or a vector of the same length as m1.
sd2 A vector of standard deviations under H_2. Must be a single number (equal standard deviation under all populations), or a vector of the same length as m2.
scale A number specifying the prior scale.
bound1 A number. The boundary above which BF12 favors H_1.
bound2 A number. The boundary below which BF12 favors H_2.
datasets A number. The number of datasets to compute the error probabilities.
nsamp A number. The number of prior or posterior samples to determine the fit and complexity.

#Output Obtained by Bayes_Sampsize

Sample size	Type 1 error	Type 2 error
46.00000000	0.08000000	0.17000000
Decision error	**Indecision error**	**Median BF12 under H1**
0.12500000	0.00000000	0.09078999

2.9.3 NPHMC

This Sample Size Calculating package is used for the Proportional Hazards Mixture having cure or without cure Model

#Sample Size Calculation for PH Mixture Cure Model and Standard PH Model

```
library("NPHMC")
NPHMC(power=0.90,alpha=0.05,accrualtime=3,
followuptime=4,p=0.5,accrualdist="uniform",
hazardratio=2/2.5,oddsratio=2.25,pi0=0.1,
survdist="exp",k=1,lambda0=0.5)
```

```
#Output on NPHMC

At alpha = 0.05 and power = 0.9 :
PH Mixture Cure Model: n = 429
Standard PH Model: n = 908
```

2.9.4   PowerTOST

This package is used for calculating the Power and Sample Size for (Bio) Equivalence Studies. It can be obtained by two and one-sided t-tests.

```
#Power and Sample Size Calculation for (Bio)Equivalence Studies

library("PowerTOST")
power.TOST(CV = 0.25, n = 24)
```

```
#Power Calculation for the 2 × 2 Cross-Over Design with 24 Subjects
and CV 25%

0.7391155
```

2.9.5   SampleSize4ClinicalTrials

This pacakge is used to calculating sample size for Means and Proportion in Phase III Clinical trials. Different ressearch design can be performed by this package. Research design like: (1) Testing for equality, (2) Superiority trial, (3) Non-inferiority trial, and (4) Equivalence trial. Now performed sample size calcuation by comparison of Means and Proportions separately.

```
#Sample Size Calculation by SampleSize4ClinicalTrials Package

library("SampleSize4ClinicalTrials")
Calculation of Means
ssc_meancomp(design = 3L, ratio = 1, alpha = 0.05, power = 0.8, sd
= 0.1, theta = 0, delta = -0.05)
Treatment Control
50          50

Calculation of Proportion
ssc_propcomp(design = 4L, ratio = 1, alpha = 0.05, power = 0.8, p1
= 0.75, p2 = 0.80, delta = 0.2)
Treatment Control
133         133
```

```
#Inputs Required for SampleSize4ClinicalTrials Package
```

design=The design of the clinical trials=1L.
Testing for equality=2L.
Superiority trial=3L.
Non-inferiority trial=4L.
Equivalence trial.
ratio=The ratio between the number of subjects in the treatment arm
and that in the control arm.
alpha=Type I error rate.
power=Statistical power of the test (1-type II error rate).
p1=The true mean response rate of the treatment arm.
p2=The true mean response rate of the control arm.
delta=The prespecified superiority, non-inferiority or equivalence
margin sample.

2.9.6   SSRMST

The sample size calculation by Restricted Mean Survival Time is possible to compute. It helps to calculate the sample size based on the difference in Restricted Mean Survival Time.

```
#SSRMST I

library("SSRMST")
ac_rate=The Accrual rate is the number of patients
per unit time. ac_period=The Accrual period as the time point at
last accrual.
ac_number=The Accrual number of accrual patients.
tot_time=The Total study time as the time point
at last follow-up.
tau Truncation is the time point to calculate RMSTs.
shape0, shape1 Shape parameters for the Weibull
distribution in
both the control (arm0) and the
treatment (arm1).
ac_rate=15
ac_period=35
tot_time = 510
tau = 500
scale0 = 7000
scale1 = 7000
margin = 10
a=ssrmst(ac_rate=ac_rate,ac_period=
ac_period, tot_time=tot_time,
tau=tau, scale0=scale0, scale1=scale1,
margin=margin, ntest=20)
print(a)
```

```
#Result of SSRMST I
```

Non-inferiority test

	Total	arm0	arm1
Sample size	524	262	262
Expected number of events	35	17	18
Power (separate)			
0.2			
Power (pooled)			
0.2			

2.9.7   powerSurvEpi

```
#Power Calculation for the Survival Analysis
```

```
library("powerSurvEpi")
ssizeEpi.default(power = 0.80, theta = 2, p = 0.39, psi = 0.505,
rho2 = 0.132^2, alpha = 0.05)
139
```

```
#Inputs Required for PowerSurvEpi Package
```

```
library("powerSurvEpi")
power=postulated power.
theta=postulated hazard ratio.
p=proportion of subjects taking value one for the covariate of interest.
psi=proportion of subjects died of the disease of interest.
rho2=square of the correlation between the covariate of interest and
the other covariate.
alpha=type I error rate.
```

2.9.8   SampleSizeMeans

This package is useful to obtain the normal means. Several functions are available to calculate the sample size by Bayesian approach. For example, "mu.acc" function is used to obtain the given coverage probability on average for a posterior credible interval of fixed length for a normal mean.

```
#SampleSizeMeans I

library("SampleSizeMeans").
mu.acc(len, alpha, beta, n0, level=0.95).
len    is the desired fixed length of the posterior
credible interval for the mean.
alpha is the First parameter of the Gamma prior density
for the precision (reciprocal of the variance).
beta is the second parameter of the Gamma prior density
for the precision (reciprocal of the variance).
n0 is the prior sample size equivalent for the mean.
level is the desired average coverage probability of the
posterior credible interval (e.g.,0.95).
#Calculated Sample Size#
mu.acc(len=0.2, alpha=2, beta=2, n0=50)
[1] 721
```

Similarly, sample size can be determined by the single normal mean using the Average Length Criterion. The function is "mu.alc". If the variance is known, then sample size is calculated by mixed of Bayesian and likelihood approach with "mu.mbl.varknown" function.

```
#SampleSizeMeans II

library("SampleSizeMeans")
mu.mbl.varknown(len, lambda, level = 0.95)
len    is the desired total length of the posterior.
credible   interval for the mean.
lambda is the known precision(reciprocal of variance).
level is the desired coverage probability of the
posterior credible interval (e.g., 0.95).
#Calculated Sample Size#
mu.mbl.varknown(len=0.2, lambda=1/4)
[1] 1537
```

Other R packages like samplesizelogisticcasecontrol,coprimary,CRTSize, EurosarcBayes,and longpower are also usefulfor sample size calculation. These are dedicated packages for sample size calculation for the clinical trial.

Chapter 3

Study Design-I

Abstract

It is preferred to define suitable statistical models for dose-response modeling. It is used as consistent by the relevant biological process with a specific case. The natural process, cell growth and biomarker changes or covariates with response variable is required under consideration. Mostly, dose-response models are curve fitting practice. Curve fitting can be performed by conventional or Bayesian approaches. This chapter is dedicated toward the application of the Bayesian technique in early phase oncology trial. Oncology trial's drugs are considered for humans with a small number of participants. The primary objective of any initial phase clinical trial is to explore the safety of a drug. Therefore, finalize the effective dose of medicine by looking acceptability on pharmacokinetics, and pharmacodynamics principle. Phase I studies are dedicated to safe-effective treatment. Oncology drugs come with a toxic agent. Phase I trial patients are cancer patients for those standard therapies failed to respond. Phase I dose-escalation method is explained with Open-BUGS. Further, the continual reassessment method is detailed by Bayesian and illustrated with an example. The model-based designs for determining the maximum tolerated dose is explained. Packages available in R for dose selection modeling is detailed.

3.1 Introduction

The Bayesian technique is prominent methodology in data science. Data science is inevitable in clinical research. So Bayesian merged tremendously in the clinical trials well. Study design, sample size calculation, and statistical analysis have emerged with the Bayesian technique. The approach to analyzing data in Bayesian is different from the classical approach. Recent computation advancement helped to incorporate Bayesian in clinical trials. It also helped to upgrade data analysis practice. Oncology research is involved with time-to-event outcomes (i.e., death). Data analysis with survival analysis

31

is not straight forward. In the presence of missing or incomplete information, it becomes more complicated. Bayesian helps to overcome different challenges. Recently, Bayesian approach is considered in several clinical trial study design. The adoption of probability is different in the Bayesian technique. The evidence-based probability plays a role in Bayesian. It helps to upgrade the proportion of uncertainty in data analysis logic. The prior information is required to incorporate. The literature review is required to upgrade the prior information. Aim of this chapter is to a show about different study design with Bayesian for oncology clinical trials.

3.2 Bayesian in Early Phase Oncology Trial

This chapter is dedicated toward the application of the Bayesian technique in early phase oncology trial. Oncology trial's drugs are considered for humans with a small number of participants. The primary objective of any early phase clinical trial is to explore the safety of a drug. Therefore, finalize the effective dose of a drug by looking acceptability on pharmacokinetics, and pharmacodynamics principle. Phase I studies are dedicated to the safe-effective dose. Oncology drugs come with a toxic agent. Phase I trial patients are cancer patients for those standard therapies failed to respond. Conventionally it is assumed that a higher drug dose will be an effective dose. Perhaps, the highest dose in oncology is decided based on a maximum tolerable dose (MTD) for cancer patients. The MTD is defined based on the dose-escalation procedure. The occurrence of severe toxicities in the first cycle of cancer therapy is defined as dose-limiting toxicities (DLTs). It is believed that the probability of toxicity and efficacy both incline with a higher dose. Hence, the objective is to define the MTD. Dose escalation study is performed with a pre-defined sample size. The increment and decrement procedure are also an important component to define MTD. The drug doses can be inclined as 10 mg, 20 mg, and 40 mg scheme. Sometimes drug comes with the non-toxic element and 50% or 25% increment of dose schemes are carried. Conventionally, the drug dose in phase I trial is defined by the rule-based. The model-based method is also suitable in another scenario. We will show a different methodology to define toxicity.

3.2.1 Rule-based designs

The rule-based design stands with prespecified dose description. In the absence of toxicity, the escalation step is carried. Similarly, in the presence of toxicity dose de-escalation. This rule-based procedure is performed with (I) 3+ 3 design, (II) Pharmacologically guided dose escalation, and (III) Accelerated titration design respectively.

3.2.1.1 3+3 design

This design is free from statistical modeling. Prespecified doses are delivered bases on the Fibonacci sequence. The absence of toxicity is called the success of a dose. The step toward a higher/lower dose is decided based on the success/failure of a dose level. A cohort of 3 patients is considered with the specified initial dose and thereafter proceed. The algorithm of this design given below.

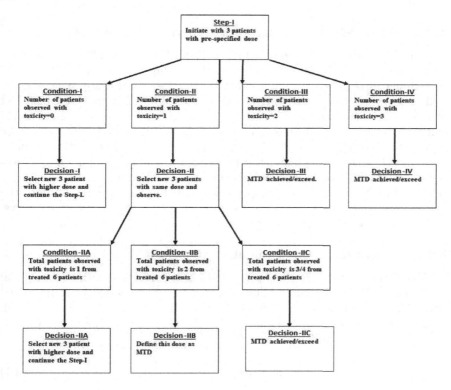

FIGURE 3.1: Flowchart of 3+3 design.

3.2.1.2 Pharmacologically guided dose escalation

This type of study useful before to carry the 3+3 design . The specific dose to start the 3+3 design can be determined by pharmacologically guided dose escalation (PGDE) design. The pharmacokinetic data are captured for each patient to define the dose level. The plasma exposure concentration is determined by pre-defined concentration-time area under the ROC curve (AUC). The 3+3 design is carried after reaching the prespecified AUC.

3.2.1.3   Accelerated titration designs

This accelerated titration designs (ATD) is an extension of the 3+3 design. It helps to reduce exposure to toxic doses to the next patient. One patient not achieved MTD is exposed with an escalated dose to establish the MTD. In this design, the same patient may be exposed to multiple doses. It also helps to treat a patient as cumulatively higher doses. However, this design only concentrates on early toxicity, not long-term toxicity.

3.2.2   Model-based designs for determining the MTD

An alternative to the rule-based methods for finding the MTD is to assume that there is a monotonic dose-response relationship between the dose and the probability of DLT for patients treated at that dose. In this approach, a dose-toxicity curve as well as the TTL are explicitly defined. The goal for the phase I clinical trial is, through treating patients in a dose escalation fashion, to seek a suitable quantile of the dose-toxicity curve; specifically, a dose that will induce a probability of DLT at a specified target toxicity level. This method is most conveniently carried out under the Bayesian framework. Simple one- or two-parameter parametric models are often used to characterize the dose-toxicity relationship, with the Bayesian posterior distribution used to estimate the parameters. These designs use all the data to model the dose-toxicity curve, and provide a credible interval for the MTD at the end of the trial.

3.2.2.1   Continual reassessment method (CRM)

The Bayesian technique is a phase I study is performed with the continual reassessment method (CRM). The dose and toxicity measurement are linked with statistical modeling. There are different models like the logistics model, tangent model, and power model. The probability of dose toxicity is defined as $p(d)$. The model is defined as

$$\text{Logistic: p(d)} = \frac{\exp(3 + ad)}{1 + \exp(3 + ad)} \tag{3.1}$$

$$\text{Hyperbolic tangent } p(d) = [(tanh(d) + 1)/2]^a = [\frac{\exp}{\exp + \exp(-d)}]^a \tag{3.2}$$

$$\text{Power}: p(d) = d^{exp(a)} \tag{3.3}$$

The parameter (a) is requried to estimate. The likelihood to obtaint the posterior estimate of a is defined as

$$L(a; d, y) \prod_{i=1}^{n} p(d_i)^{y_i} [1 - p(d_i)]^{1-y_i} \tag{3.4}$$

Now d_i and y_i are the dose level and toxicity outcome for patient i, and where $y_i = 1$ if a DLT is observed and $y_i = 0$ if not. The algorithm to perform the CRM design is given in the following text.

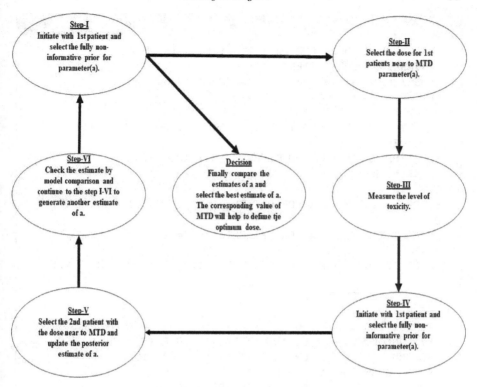

FIGURE 3.2: Flowchart of continual reassessment design.

3.3   Study Design Package Using R

```
Phase I Dose-Escalation Method Using R

library("bcrm")
p.tox0 <- c(0.05, 0.10, 0.20, 0.30)
dose.label <- c(5, 10, 15, 25)
bcrm(stop = list(nmax = 28), p.tox0 = p.tox0,
dose = dose.label,ff = "power",
prior.alpha = list(1, 1, 1), target.tox = 0.30,start = 1)
```

R Output

```
RECOMMENDED DOSE FOR PATIENTS 1 to 3 IS: 5
ENTER DOSE FOR PATIENTS 1 to 3
POSSIBLE CHOICES ARE 5 10 15 25 40 50 60
EITHER:
a) HIT 'RETURN' TO ACCEPT RECOMMENDATION
b) TYPE ANOTHER POSSIBLE DOSE AND HIT 'RETURN' TO USE
ANOTHER DOSE
c) TYPE '0' AND HIT 'RETURN' TO EXIT AND RETURN
CURRENT RESULTS)
5
ENTER TOXICITY DATA FOR PATIENT 1 (1 = TOX, 0 = NO TOX):
0
ENTER TOXICITY DATA FOR PATIENT 2 (1 = TOX, 0 = NO TOX):
0
ENTER TOXICITY DATA FOR PATIENT 3 (1 = TOX, 0 = NO TOX):
0
         ENTERED VALUES:
DOSE ... 5
TOXICITIES ... 0 0 0
HIT 'RETURN' IF OK OR ANY OTHER KEY TO ENTER NEW VALUES
RECOMMENDED DOSE FOR PATIENTS 4 to 6 IS: 10
ENTER DOSE FOR PATIENTS 4 to 6
POSSIBLE CHOICES ARE 5 10 15 25 40 50 60
EITHER:
a) HIT 'RETURN' TO ACCEPT RECOMMENDATION
b) TYPE ANOTHER POSSIBLE DOSE AND HIT 'RETURN' TO USE
ANOTHER DOSE
c) TYPE '0' AND HIT 'RETURN' TO EXIT AND RETURN CURRENT
 RESULTS)
```

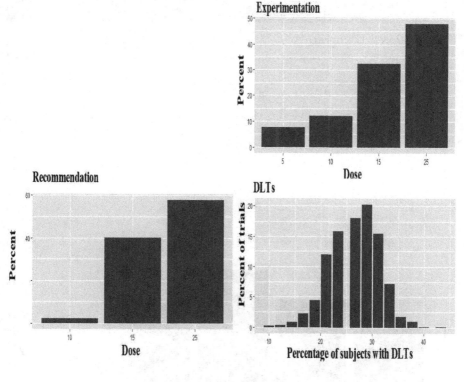

FIGURE 3.3: Phase I dose-escalation method using R.

```
Dose-Escalation to Decide the DLT with R

library("bcrm")
dose <- c(1,2.5,5,10,15,20,25,30,40,50,75,100,150,200,250)
p.tox0 <- c(0.010, 0.015, 0.020, 0.025, 0.030, 0.040, 0.050,
0.100, 0.170, 0.300, 0.400, 0.500, 0.650, 0.800, 0.900)
## Data from the first 5 cohorts of 18 patients
data <- data.frame(patient=1:18, dose=rep(c(1:4, 7),
c(3, 4, 5, 4, 2)), tox=rep(0:1, c(16, 2)))
## Target toxicity level
target.tox <- 0.30
## A 1-parameter power model is used, with standardised
doses calculated using
## the plug-in prior median
## Prior for alpha is lognormal with mean 0 (on log scale)
## and standard deviation 1.34 (on log scale)
Power.LN.bcrm <- bcrm(stop=list(nmax=18), data=data,
p.tox0=p.tox0, dose=dose, ff="power",
prior.alpha=list(3, 0, 1.34^2),
target.tox=target.tox, constrain=FALSE,
sdose.calculate="median", pointest="mean")
```

R Output to Finalized the Dose

plot(Power.LN.bcrm)

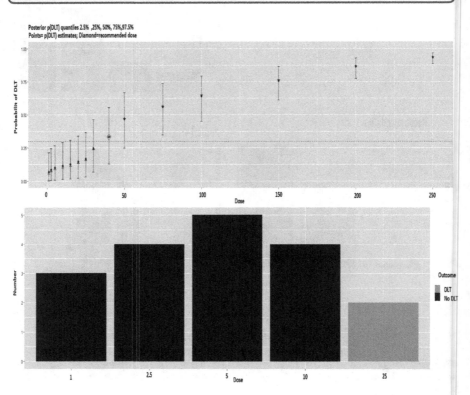

FIGURE 3.4: Dose-escalation cancer trial of DLT.

Chapter 4

Study Design-II

Abstract

It is a difficult task to decide optimal study design for phase II study. Sometimes, it becomes more complicated while work with new molecular targeted agents. as a result, phase III gets failed. It raises the issue that several agents to be tested with the increasing complexity and cost. Simultaneously, the study design is expected to be robust and efficient. This chapter is dedicated to a phase II study design. Different study designs are considered to perform phase II study. Similarly, different types of outcomes may arise in phase II study as binary and continuous outcomes. Results observed with binary or continuous are illustrated. Likewise, the sample size is another issue for the phase II study design. Sample size determination procedure also elaborated. Different R packages required to perform phase II study with the Bayesian approach are explained. Example are presented with prior value, likelihood and posterior estimates generation. This chapter will help to perform a Phase II study in oncology domains.

4.1   Introduction

Phase II oncology trials are performed to decide a trial can be conducted in massive or not. The primary endpoint in oncology trial is tumor size reduction. Similarly, the disease progression both is critical endpoints in Phase-II clinical trials. Drugs used in oncology are cytostatic. The cytostatic drug destroys the tumor cells and increases survival. The effect of the cytostatic drug is measured by progression-free survival. However, the tumor progression and tumor shrinkage both are anatomical burdens of the tumor. The tumor size reduction is decided based on the Response Evaluation Criteria in Solid Tumors (RECIST). There are clinicians from academia and industry, image specialist, statistician and another subject expert to as RECIST Working Group. The RECIST guideline is routinely updated. The target of Cytostatic drugs is molecularly targeted agents (MTA). The control on MTA helps to prolong the survival. The solid tumor classified as progressive disease (PD), partial responses (PR), stable disease (SD) or complete responses (CR).The terms PD and SD stand with treatment failure. Similarly, treatment success as CR and PR. Jointly the PR and CR patients are defined as the objective response rate (ORR). The proportion of patients under disease control are defined as the disease control rate (DCR). It is better to not bring Phase II patients into Phase III due to the occurrence of the substantial risk of toxicity or death. The measurement of toxicity requires to take in Phase II trial design. The combined inference about treatment success is decided by (I) change in tumor size, (II) occurrence of new lesions, and (III) death/relapse. The treatment failure is defined as a dichotomous endpoint (died or not). But the reduction in tumor size is measured as continuous (i.e., the amount of tumor shrinkage). Perhaps, the tumor shrinkage can be classified into a dichotomous category by predefined threshold reduction. The consolidated endpoint is measured by continuous and binary components. The challenge is to estimate the different probability and compare the uncertainty of the estimates by confidence interval (CI).

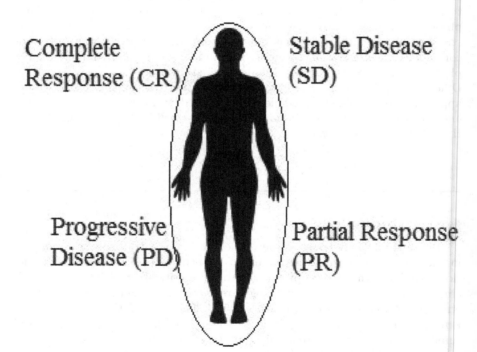

FIGURE 4.1: Disease progression cycle.

4.2 Methods

4.2.1 Estimating treatment success

Suppose that the proportion of tumor shrinkage is assumed as 20%, and these patients are free from toxicity or death. A total of n patients are allocated to the treatment under consideration. The measurements are taken as t_{1i}, t_{2i} and t_{3i}. Now $D_{1i} = 1$ if patients "i" fails due to other reason and $D_{2i} = 1$ if fails occurs during the two measurement. The log tumor size ratio is defined as

$$(y_{1i}, y_{2i}) = (\log(\frac{z_{1i}}{z_{0i}}), \log(\frac{z_{2i}}{z_{0i}})) \tag{4.1}$$

Further, the tumor shrinkage model is defined with bivariate distribution

$$(y_{1i}, y_{2i})^T | z_{i0} \approx N((\mu_{1i}, \mu_{2i})^T, \sum) \tag{4.2}$$

where

$$\mu_{1i} = \alpha + \gamma z_{i0}, \mu_{2i} = \beta + \gamma z_{i0} \tag{4.3}$$

If non-shrinkage tumor size is intermediately unmeasured, then it can be treated as missing at random (MAR). The model can be estimated by the linear model. The probability of non-shrinkage failure before the interim measurement is presented as a probability of $D_{i1} = 1$. If non-shrinkage tumor size is intermediately unmeasured, then it can be treated as missing at random (MAR). The model can be estimated by the linear model. The probability of non-shrinkage failure before the interim measurement is presented as a probability of $D_{i1} = 1$. Logistics Model is useful for both model

$$\text{Logit}(P(D_{i1} = 1)|Z_{i0}) = \alpha D_1 + \gamma D_1 z_{i0} \tag{4.4}$$

$$\text{Logit}(P(D_{i2} = 1|D_{i1} = 0, Z_{i0}, Z_{i1}) = \alpha D_2 + \gamma D_2 z_{i1} \tag{4.5}$$

Let the covariance matrix is $\sum$. The vector parameter θ is used to represent the tumor shrinkage and non-shrinkage model. The probability of treatment success for the ith patients with baseline tumor size z_{oi} is as follows:

$$P(S_i = 1|z_{0i}, \theta) = \int_{-\infty}^{\infty} P(S_i = 1|z_{0i}, y_{1i}, y_{2i}, \theta) f_{Y_1, Y_2}(y_{1i}, y_{2i}; \theta) dy_{1i} dy_{2i} \tag{4.6}$$

$$P(S_i = 1|z_{0i}, \theta) = \int_{-\infty}^{\log(0.7)} \int_{-\infty}^{\infty} \tag{4.7}$$
$$P(D_{1i} = 0|z_{0i}, \theta) P(D_{2i} = 0|D_{1i} = 0, z_{0i}, y_{1i}; \theta) dy_{1i} dy_{2i}$$

The pdf of the bivaraite distribution is defined as $f_{Y_1, Y_2}(y_{1i}, y_{2i}; \theta)$.

The mean of treatment success is presented as

$$\hat{P}(S = 1|\theta) = \sum_{i=1}^{n} \frac{P(S_i = 1|z_{0i}, \theta)}{n} \tag{4.8}$$

and estimated as $\hat{P}(S = 1|\hat{\theta})$.

The confidence interval for $l(\theta)$ is obtained through variance of $l(\hat{\theta})$ as

$$\text{var}(l(\hat{\theta})) \approx (\nabla l(\hat{\theta}))^T \text{var}(\hat{\theta})(\nabla l(\hat{\theta})) \tag{4.9}$$

The delta method is useful to obtain the estimate.

4.2.2   Treatment difference testing

Suppose there are $2n$ patients allocated to two arms by n. The tumor shrinkage is defined as

$$(y_{i1}, y_{i2})^T | t_i, z_{i0} \sim N((\mu_{11}, \mu_{2i})^T, \textstyle\sum) \tag{4.10}$$

The ith patients 1st observation is determined as y_{i1}. The mean response of ith patients 1st measurement is defined as

$$\mu_{1i} = \mu + \beta_1 t_i + \gamma z_{i0} \tag{4.11}$$

$$\mu_{2i} = \mu + \delta + \beta_2 t_i + \gamma z_{i0} \tag{4.12}$$

the treatment is defined as t_i for the ith patient.

Now the tumor non-shrinkage model is defined as

$$\text{Logit}(P(D_{i1} = 1|t_i, z_{i0})) = \alpha_{D_1} + \beta_{D_1} t_i + \gamma_{D_1} z_{i0} \tag{4.13}$$

$$\text{Logit}(P(D_{i2} = 1|D_{i1} = 0, t_i, z_{i0}, z_{i1})) = \alpha_{D_2} + \beta_{D_2} t_i + \gamma_{D_2} z_{i1} \tag{4.14}$$

The probability of treatment sucess from shrinkage and non-shrinkage is defined as $P(S = 1|t, z_0, \theta)$. It is reformulated as

$$m(\theta) = \sum_{i=1}^{2n} \frac{P(S_i = 1|t = 1, z_{0i}, \theta) - P(S_i = 1|t = 0, z_{0i}, \theta)}{2n} \tag{4.15}$$

The term θ is used as vector parameter and it can be formulated as

$$m(\theta) = \sum_{i=1}^{2n} \frac{P(S_i = 1|t = 1, z_{0i}, \theta) - P(S_i = 1|t = 0, z_{0i}, \theta)}{2n} \tag{4.16}$$

The estimate of $m(\theta)$ is determined as $m(\hat{\theta})$. Th e delta method is useful to obtain the estimate of $m(\theta)$. The Wald statistic is performed to obtain the test statistics.

4.3   Illustration with Bayesian Using R

```
# Different Prior Distribution Assumption

library("trialr") # Call trialr libary in R#
library("Rcpp")# Call Rcpp libary in R#
priors <- list(alpha_mean = 0, alpha_sd = 1,
beta_mean = 0, beta_sd = 1,gamma_mean = 0, gamma_sd = 1,
sigma_mean = 0, sigma_sd = 1,omega_lkj_eta = 1,
alpha_d1_mean=0,alpha_d1_sd=1,gamma_d1_mean=0,gamma_d1_sd=1,
alpha_d2_mean=0,alpha_d2_sd=1,gamma_d2_mean=0,gamma_d2_sd=1)
#generate data named as "prior" #
#with different distribution assumption#
library("trialr")
N <- 50 # Assigned sample size 50 to generate data#
sigma <- 1 # seed value assumption about varaince#
delta1 <- -0.356 # seed value assumption about delta#
mu <- c(0.5 × delta1, delta1) # generate mean value#
Sigma = matrix(c(0.5 × sigma^2, 0.5 × sigma^2, 0.5 × sigma^2,
sigma^2),ncol = 2)
alphaD <- -1.5
gammaD <- 0
set.seed(123456)
y <- MASS::mvrnorm(n = N, mu, Sigma)
z0 <- runif(N, min = 5, max = 10)
z1 <- exp(y[, 1]) × z0
z2 <- exp(y[, 2]) × z0
d1 <- rbinom(N, size = 1, prob = gtools::inv.logit(alphaD
+ gammaD × z0))
d2 <- rbinom(N, size = 1, prob = gtools::inv.logit(alphaD
+ gammaD × z1))
tumor_size <- data.frame(z0, z1, z2) # Sizes in cm
non_shrinkage_failure <- data.frame(d1, d2)
fit <- stan_augbin(tumor_size, non_shrinkage_failure,
prior_params=priors,model ='2t-1a', seed = 123)
fit
```

```
Sampling for Model 'AugBin2T1A' with (Chain 1)


Chain 1:
Chain 1: Gradient evaluation took 0 seconds
Chain 1: 1000 transitions using 10 leapfrog steps
per transition would take 0 seconds.
Chain 1: Adjust your expectations accordingly!
Chain 1:
Chain 1:
Chain 1: Iteration:    1 / 2000 [  0%]  (Warmup)
Chain 1: Iteration:  200 / 2000 [ 10%]  (Warmup)
Chain 1: Iteration:  400 / 2000 [ 20%]  (Warmup)
Chain 1: Iteration:  600 / 2000 [ 30%]  (Warmup)
Chain 1: Iteration:  800 / 2000 [ 40%]  (Warmup)
Chain 1: Iteration: 1000 / 2000 [ 50%]  (Warmup)
Chain 1: Iteration: 1001 / 2000 [ 50%]  (Sampling)
Chain 1: Iteration: 1200 / 2000 [ 60%]  (Sampling)
Chain 1: Iteration: 1400 / 2000 [ 70%]  (Sampling)
Chain 1: Iteration: 1600 / 2000 [ 80%]  (Sampling)
Chain 1: Iteration: 1800 / 2000 [ 90%]  (Sampling)
Chain 1: Iteration: 2000 / 2000 [100%]  (Sampling)
Chain 1:
Chain 1:   Elapsed Time: 5.849 seconds (Warm-up)
Chain 1:                 4.818 seconds (Sampling)
Chain 1:                 10.667 seconds (Total)
Chain 1:
```

```
Sampling for Model 'AugBin2T1A' with (Chain 2)

Chain 2:
Chain 2: Gradient evaluation took 0 seconds
Chain 2: 1000 transitions using 10 leapfrog steps
per transition would take 0 seconds.
Chain 2: Adjust your expectations accordingly!
Chain 2:
Chain 2:
Chain 2: Iteration:    1 / 2000 [  0%]  (Warmup)
Chain 2: Iteration:  200 / 2000 [ 10%]  (Warmup)
Chain 2: Iteration:  400 / 2000 [ 20%]  (Warmup)
Chain 2: Iteration:  600 / 2000 [ 30%]  (Warmup)
Chain 2: Iteration:  800 / 2000 [ 40%]  (Warmup)
Chain 2: Iteration: 1000 / 2000 [ 50%]  (Warmup)
Chain 2: Iteration: 1001 / 2000 [ 50%]  (Sampling)
Chain 2: Iteration: 1200 / 2000 [ 60%]  (Sampling)
Chain 2: Iteration: 1400 / 2000 [ 70%]  (Sampling)
Chain 2: Iteration: 1600 / 2000 [ 80%]  (Sampling)
Chain 2: Iteration: 1800 / 2000 [ 90%]  (Sampling)
Chain 2: Iteration: 2000 / 2000 [100%]  (Sampling)
Chain 2:
Chain 2:  Elapsed Time: 5.702 seconds (Warm-up)
Chain 2:                14.104 seconds (Sampling)
Chain 2:                19.806 seconds (Total)
Chain 2:
```

```
Inference for Stan Model: AugBin2T1A

4 chains, each with iter=2000; warmup=1000; thin=1;

post-warmup draws per chain=1000, total post-warmup
draws=4000.
            Mean    SE    SD    2.5%    97.5%    neff    R
alpha       0.07   0.01  0.44   -0.78   0.94     2008    1
beta       -0.11   0.01  0.44   -0.97   0.75     2122    1
gamma      -0.02   0.00  0.06   -0.14  -0.09     2135    1
Omega11     1.00   NaN   0.00    1.00   1.00     NaN    NaN
Omega1,2    0.73   0.00  0.07    0.58   0.84     2733    1
Omega2,1    0.73   0.00  0.07    0.58   0.84     2733    1
Omega2,2    1.00   0.00  0.00    1.00   1.00     3974    1
sigma1      0.74   0.00  0.07    0.62   0.90     3058    1
sigma2      1.04   0.00  0.10    0.86   1.27     3097    1
alphaD1    -0.22   0.02  0.85   -1.90   1.44     2734    1
gammaD1    -0.15   0.00  0.13   -0.40   0.10     2861    1
alphaD2    -0.30   0.01  0.52   -1.33   0.72     3288    1
gammaD2    -0.08   0.00  0.06   -0.23   0.03     3021    1
 For each parameter, neff is a crude measure of effective
 sample size,and Rhat is the potential scale reduction
 factor on split chains (at convergence, R=1$).
```

4.4   Discussion

The proposed methods work in combination with binary and continuous outcomes. It is suited well in phase II cancer research. The method compatible one decision about binary and another response about continuous outcomes. The sample size determination is a phase II clinical trial is a significant issue. Conventionally study design is required to calculate the sample size. It can be specified that any Phase II study planned with 50 sample size can be accommodated with the pre-specified methodology.

Chapter 5

Optimum Biological Dose Selection

Abstract

The biomarker is a realistic indicator to explore angiogenesis in cancer. Recently, Subtoxic doses of chemotherapy are administered and defined as Metronomic Chemotherapy (MC). Now set the best effective treatment in MC is a challenging task. This chapter is elaborated about dose fixation by looking biomarker level. The dose could help to maintain the desired level of the biomarker as the optimum biological dose (OBD). We presented the Bayesian algorithm to determine the OBD. The curve fitting procedure is illustrated in OpenBUGS to determine the OBD. This work is explored by looking at the performance of one surrogate marker toward influencing the disease outcome. Disease outcome is defined as time-to-event outcomes. Conventional, time-to-event methodology like Kaplan-Meier estimates are elaborated. Similarly, the treatment outcome is classified as a dose that is suitable to control the OBD. In this chapter, theoretical explanation about Toxicity profile testing, Logistic Response Model and Quadratic Logistic Design are detailed with Bayesian illustration. The illustration will help to determine the best dose by looking at the posterior estimates of regression coefficients. Similarly, model suitability is explained by standard deviation and model selection criteria.

5.1 Introduction

The maximum dose of the effective drug within the tolerable limit is called the maximum tolerated dose (MTD). Conventionally, it assumed that increased dose is effective. The best effective dose concluded by one level below the tolerable highest dose [3, 4, 5]. Metronomic chemotherapy (MC) emerges as a therapeutic option in medical oncology [6, 7, 8]. Sometimes, conventional chemotherapy becomes resistant [8, 9, 10]. Development of chemoresistance is a common problem [11]. The alternative of high-dose chemotherapy stands with Metronomic chemotherapy (MC). The MC causes less severe side effects than standard chemotherapy. The MC is marked as low-dose chemotherapy.

47

Now the determination of best effective dose in MC is a challenging task. The predefined biomarker is considered to represent the disease status. The threshold value of a biomarker is required to define the disease status. Thereafter the task is to explore that the MC is most effective to maintain the biomarker's desired value. The MC is decided by the optimum biological dose (OBD)[12]. In this chapter, we will explore the Bayesian approach to decided the low dose of chemotherapy.

5.2 Illustration with Head and Neck Cancer Data

Establishing a biomarker for cancer is a difficult task. Unless biomarker is established, it is challenging to establish the best effective metronomic dose. We will illustrate the methodology with simulated data. A simulation study was carried to explore the OBD and check the MC performance. The skewed distribution was used to obtain the head and neck cancer (HNC) data. The circulating endothelial cell (CEC) is considered as a biomarker. The repeatedly measured CEC is controlled within the desired level or not is considered as an outcome of dose. The prior mean 114 and standard deviation 15 are considered to generated CEC measurement. A total of 4 doses named as dose 1, dose 2 dose 3 and dose 4 are presented. Data is generated for a total of 220 patients. Persons alive status is presented as 0 or 1. the solid tumor size is generated from (mean 4.0 cm, SD 2). histological grading is measured as (well, moderate and poor)were generated randomly for a total of 220 patients and merged with the excel sheet. The survival representation is provided by the Kaplan-Meier curve on progression-free survival in Figure 5.4. Relapse is considered an event. A total of five follow-up visits observations for CEC and tumor size were assumed to be distributed with a normal distribution. Different time points are assumed as t_1, t_2, t_3, t_4, t_5 . Corresponding mean of CEC is assumed as 124, 128, 135, 126, and 120 respectively. Censored distribution about duration of survival was obtained from a hazard rate of 0.0003 with approximately 45% censored observations.

5.3 Toxicity Profile Testing

Suppose the specific dose is defined as d_j from a set of doses i.e.$(d_1, ..., d_J)$. Now a total of n patients are exposed with dose level j. However, a low dose of chemotherapy is free from toxicity. However, we show a provision about measure the toxicity profile in addition to the efficacy level.

Now the q_j is presented as the toxicity of dose level d_j. A total of x_j patients are observed with toxicity occurrence with a specific dose of d_j. The prior assumption about d_j is obtained as

$$x_j \sim \text{binom}(n_j, q_j) \tag{5.1}$$

Probability of toxicity q_j is assumed as

$$q_j \sim \text{beta}(a, b) \tag{5.2}$$

The hyperparameters are a and b. maximum tolerable toxicity range is ϕ. Patients exposed to dose level are presumed as j is x_j. Posterior distribution about $\Pr(q_j > \phi | \eta_j, x_j)$ is obtained to perform the model diagnostic among different doses d_j.

$$A = \{ j : \bar{P}r(q_j > \phi | \eta_j, x_j) < C_\tau, j = 1, \ldots J \} \tag{5.3}$$

The prespecified dose limit is C_τ with specific toxicity level. The term C_τ can be defined as a tolerable limit or threshold limit. It helps to protect patients from the occurrence of over toxicity. A small prior assumption of a, b are used with threshold value as $\text{Beta}(\phi; a, b) = 1 - C_\tau + \delta$. The limit of δ is captured with a small positive number 0.5.

5.4 Logistic Response Model

The logistics model is defined below. The biomarker is considered as CEC. The dose could maintain the limit of a CEC is defined as OBD. The probability of sucess is defined as $g(p_j)$. The corresponding dose is termed as d_j. The function $f(s)$ is used to define the threshold value of OBD as

$$g(p_j) = \beta_1 + \beta_2 d_j \tag{5.4}$$

The predefined dose of OBD is determined as $[c_1, c_2]$ with uniform distribution

$$f(s) = \begin{cases} \frac{1}{c_2 - c_1} & \text{if } c_1 \le s \le c_2; \\ 0 & \text{if otherwise.} \end{cases}$$

The cummulative dose is presented as p_j as

$$p_j = \int_{c_1}^{d_j} f(s)ds = \frac{d_j - c_1}{c_2 - c_1} \text{ for } c_1 \le d_j \le c_2 \tag{5.5}$$

It becomes $\beta_1 = \frac{-c_1}{c_2 - c_1}$ and $\beta_2 = \frac{1}{c_2 - c_1}$

The OBD is defined as $c_1 \leq d_j \leq c_2$. It is expected that p_j will distribut
normally as

$$p_j = \frac{1}{2\pi} \int_{-\infty}^{x} \exp[-\frac{1}{2}(\frac{s-\mu}{\sigma})^2]ds, \Phi \sim N(0,1) \tag{5.6}$$

$$\Phi^{-1}(p_j) = \beta_1 + \beta_2 d_j \tag{5.7}$$

where $\beta_1 = -\mu/\sigma$ and $\beta_2 = 1/\sigma$. The link function g is adopted with
inverse cumulative Normal probability function Φ^{-1}.

The function of OBD is defined as

$$f(s) = \frac{\beta_2 \exp(\beta_1 + \beta_2 s)}{[1 + \exp(\beta_1 + \beta_2 s)]^2} \tag{5.8}$$

so

$$p_j = \int_{-\infty}^{x} f(s)ds = \frac{exp(\beta_1 + \beta_2 d_j)}{[1 + exp(\beta_1 + \beta_2 d_j)]} \tag{5.9}$$

The link function is considered as

$$\log(\frac{p_j}{1 - p_j}) = \beta_1 + \beta_2 d_j \tag{5.10}$$

The probability of sucess due to dose label d_j is p_i. The model is defined as

$$p_j = \frac{\exp(\beta_1 + \beta_2 d_j)}{1 + \exp(\beta_1 + \beta_2 d_j)} \tag{5.11}$$

$$\log(\frac{p_j}{1 - p_j}) = \beta_1 + \beta_2 d_j \tag{5.12}$$

$$\log(1 - p_j) = -\log[1 + \exp(\beta_1 + \beta_2 d_j)] \tag{5.13}$$

If the patients size is N then the log-likelihood function can be defined as

$$l = \sum_{i=1}^{N}[y_i(\beta_1 + \beta_2 d_j) - n_i \log[1 + \exp(\beta_1 + \beta_2 d_j)] + \log\binom{n_i}{y_i}) \tag{5.14}$$

$$U_1 = \frac{\delta l}{\delta \beta_1} = \sum\{y_i - n_i[\frac{\exp(\beta_1 + \beta_2 d_i)}{1 + \exp(\beta_1 + \beta_2 d_i)}]\} = \sum(y_i - n_i p_j) \tag{5.15}$$

$$U_2 = \frac{\delta l}{\delta \beta_2} = \sum\{y_i d_j - n_i d_j[\frac{\exp(\beta_1 + \beta_2 d_j)}{1 + \exp(\beta_1 + \beta_2 d_j)}]\} \tag{5.16}$$

$$U_2 = \sum(y_i - n_i p_j) = \sum d_j(y_i - n_i p_j) \tag{5.17}$$

The information matrix is defined as

$$T = \begin{vmatrix} \sum n_i p_j(1 - p_j) & \sum n_i d_j p_j(1 - p_j) \\ \sum n_i d_j p_j(1 - p_j) & \sum n_i d_j^2 p_j(1 - p_j) \end{vmatrix}.$$

The maximum likelihood estimates is defined as

$$T^{(m-1)}b^m = I^{(m-1)}b^{(m-1)} + U^{(m-1)} \tag{5.18}$$

The number of approximation is defined as (m) and vector of estimates is given as b through with deviance function as,

$$D = 2\sum_{i=1}^{N}[y_i\log(\frac{y_i}{\hat{y}_i}) + (n_i - y_i)\log(\frac{n_i - y_i}{n_i - \hat{y}_i})] \tag{5.19}$$

5.5 Dose Selection Algorithm

Dose Selection Algorithm

The OBD of low-dose chemotherapy will be decided based on the following steps:

(I)Start to recruit a very minimal number of patients for a specific dose level j.

(II)The minimal number of patients will be defined as l.

(III)Measure the toxicity for each dose level.

(IV) Similarly, the dose level $l - 1$ will be measured.

(V) Credible interval of posterior estimates will be obtained for each dose by posterior probability distribution with $\Pr(\beta > 0|d_j)$.

(V) Now it may possible that the dose $j+1$ comes with $\Pr(\beta > 0|d_j) > C_{E1}$.

(VI)Decision about escalation will be concluded by looking dose level $\Pr(\beta > 0|d_j) < C_{E2}$ probability.

(VII) Decision about de-escalation will be concluded by dose level $\Pr(\beta > 0|d_j) < C_{E2}$, to the dose level $j - 1$.

(VIII)The next step is to continue the study with a specific dose and cover the maximum sample size.

(IX) Finally, the optimum dose will be determined by the maximum pick of the curve reached by the dose levels.

(X) The best dose will be obtained by calibration on C_{E1} and C_{E2}.

5.6   Quadratic Logistic Design

A specific dose is effective or not can be classified into binary format. Let us assume that the dose level is j and sucess of dose is p_j. The quadratic lonistic curve is defined as

$$\log(\frac{p_j}{1 - p_j}) = \alpha + \beta d_j + \gamma d_j^2, j = 1, 2, ...j \qquad (5.20)$$

Suppose there are γ_i patients treated with d_j dose from a toal of η_j. The likelihood function is $D = \{y_j, \eta_j; j = 1, ..., J\}$ with

$$L(D|\alpha, \beta, \gamma) \propto \prod_{j=1}^{J} (\frac{e^{\alpha+\beta d_j+\gamma d_j^2}}{1 + e^{\alpha+\beta d_j+\gamma d_j^2}})^{\gamma_j} (\frac{1}{1 + e^{\alpha+\beta d_j+\gamma d_j^2}})^{\eta_i-\gamma_i} \qquad (5.21)$$

The posterior estimates of the parameters will be obtained by Markov chain Monte Carlo (MCMC) method. The α is assumed with prior assumption Cauchy(0,10) distribution. Similarly, β and γ will be obtained from Cauchy(0,2.5).

TABLE 5.1: Median estimates of survival among different doses

Doses	Number at risk	Events	Median	0.95LCL	0.95UCL
d_1	249	139	50	43	58
d_2	246	130	53	49	64
d_3	246	135	49	41	57
d_4	236	122	48	42	57

TABLE 5.2: Posterior estimates of the models through measurement of surrogate marker

Mode l	Parameter	Posterior Mean	SD	HPD	DIC
	β_1	332.2	74.81	(216.9,450.1)	
Model1	β_2	-8.182	6.47	(18.56,1.942)	253.2
	σ_1	67.19	12.21	(48.25,95.6)	
	τ_1	0.00024	0.00008	(0.0001,0.0004)	
	α	679.0	2621.0	(-604.6, 10660.0)	
	β	-74.28	502.5	(-1983.0, 170.8)	
Model 2	γ	2.923	22.45	(-7.975, 87.25)	226.4
	σ_2	74.66	28.77	(47.66, 179.7)	
	τ_2	0.00021	0.00010	(0.00025,0.00043)	

TABLE 5.3: Performance of methods through the measurement of surrogate marker

Scenario	Characteristics	d_1	d_2	d_3	d_4	Overtoxic
				Dose		
Scenario 1:	Selected Probability	0.01	0.10	0.20	0.69	0
	Proportion of Patients	0.08	0.19	0.1	0.63	
Scenario 2:	Selected Probability	0.12	0.15	0.23	0.50	0
	Proportion of Patients	0.18	0.22	0.09	0.51	
Scenario 3:	Selected Probability	0.21	0.27	0.15	0.37	0.01
	Proportion of Patients	0.35	0.29	0.04	0.32	
Scenario 4:	Selected Probability	0.29	0.43	0.18	0.10	0
	Proportion of Patients	0.49	0.31	0.1	0.10	

5.7 Illustration

In this illustration, two models are provided. Results are obtained through posterior mean and standard deviation. A different scenario is prepared, and those are given in Table 5.3. It provides the scope to consider the doses and toxicity occurrences. The optimal dose can be obtained from this table. Since

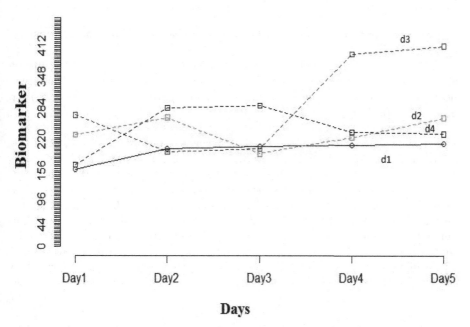

FIGURE 5.1: Different doses and biomarker value changes.

Dose and Biomarker

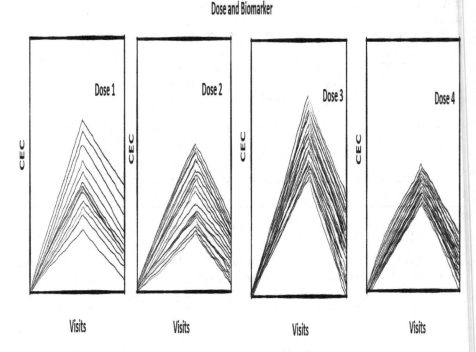

FIGURE 5.2: Biomarker changes over the visits.

the work is about low-dose chemotherapy, then the appearance of over toxicity is very minimal.

This work is presented by a simulation study. The posterior probability of efficacy and safety is presented as E and S, respectively. Suppose the marginal posterior probability of the associated parameters are defined as (σ_2 or τ_2) for S and E respectively.

The parameter S and E is linked as $\Pr(S = 1) = V * \Pr(E = 1)$. Now $V = 1$ shows that OBD through a biomarker is achieved. If $V > 1$, then the OBD of a biomarker is not achieved. Now the term σ and τ represents the relation between S and E. if there is no relation between σ_1 and τ_1 then the efficacy E could be ignored and the corresponding dose may be ignored. Now Logistic response model is defined as Model1. Similarly, Quadratic Logistic design is defined as Model 2. The additive parameters σ and τ for Model 1 is defined as σ_1 and τ_1 respectively. Similarly, Model 2 is defined as σ_2 and τ_2. In this illustration a total of 20,000 iterations with 1,000 burn-in is carried out with different fixed value of $\sigma_1, \tau_1, \sigma_2$ and τ_2 . The simulation is performed to obtain the convergence. The convergence is obtained by observing the trace

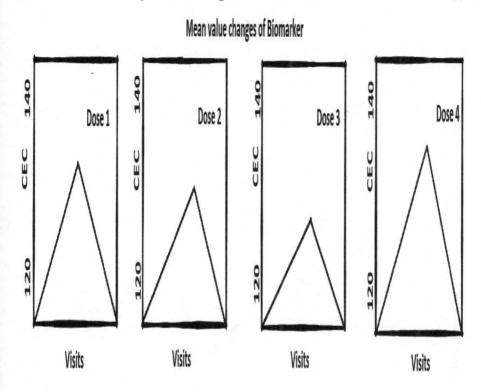

FIGURE 5.3: Mean Biomarker changes over the visits.

plots for each parameter of the model. The models are compared by Decision Information Criteria(DIC) value.

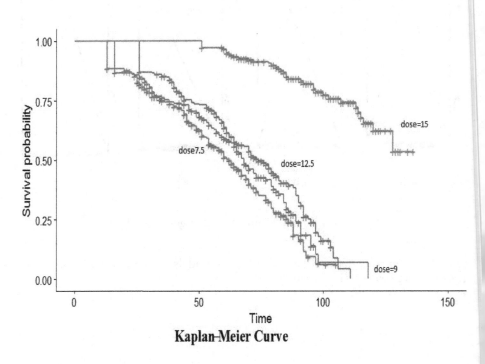

FIGURE 5.4: Dose-wise survival curve comparison.

5.8 Bayesian Dose Selection Using OpenBUGS

```
# OpenBUGS code 1

Model1
model
{
for (i in 1:20)
{
mu.dmf[i] <- beta1 + beta2 × fl[i]
dmf[i] ~ dnorm(mu.dmf[i],tau)
}
beta1 ~ dnorm(0.0,0.000001)
beta2 ~ dnorm(0.0,0.000001)
sigma1 ~ dunif(0,400)
tau1 <- 1/(sigma1×sigma1)
for (i in 1:20)
{ # calculate residuals
residual[i] <- dmf[i] - mu.dmf[i]
}
pred.mean.1.7 <- beta1 + beta2×1.7
pred.ind.1.7 ~ dnorm(pred.mean.1.7, tau1)
}
```

```
# OpenBUGS code 2

Model2
model {
for (i in 1:20)
{
mu.dmf[i] <- alpha + beta×fl[i] + gamma×fl[i]×fl[i]
# regression equation
dmf[i] ~ dnorm(mu.dmf[i],tau)
# distribution individual values
}
alpha ~ dnorm(0.0, 0.000001)
beta ~ dnorm(0.0, 0.000001)
gamma ~ dnorm(0.0, 0.000001)
sigma2 ~ dunif(0,200)
tau2 <- 1/(sigma2×sigma2)
for (i in 1:20)
{ # calculate residuals
residual[i] <- dmf[i]-mu.dmf[i]
}
pred.mean.1.7 <- alpha + beta1×1.7 + beta2×1.7×1.7
# mean prediction for fl=1.7
pred.ind.1.7 ~ dnorm(pred.mean.1.7, tau2)
# individual pred for fl=1.7
}
```

```
# OpenBUGS code 2

dmf[] fl[]
159 15
168 7.5
201 15
206 15
209 15
212 15
230 12.5
265 12.5
270 9
285 7.5
290 7.5
195 9
201 9
236 7.5
191 12.5
225 12.5
232 7.5
265 12.5
396 9
412 9
END
list(dmf=c( 159,168,201,206,209,212,230,265,
270,285,290,195,201,236,191,225,232,265,396,
412),
fl=c(15,7.5,15,15,15,15,12.5,12.5,9,7.5,
7.5,9,9,7.5,12.5,12.5,7.5,12.5,9,9))}
```

5.9 Discussion

The MC can be classified as next-generation chemotherapy [13]. It is possible to explore the performance of one surrogate marker toward influencing the disease outcome. Similarly, the treatment outcome can be classified as a dose best to control the OBD. Perhaps, it is difficult to establish the biomarker or surrogate marker.

5.10   Dose Finding Package Using R

5.10.1   DoseFinding

```
#DoseFinding package with R for samplesize determination

install.packages("DoseFinding")
library("DoseFinding")
doses <- c(0, 10, 25, 50, 100, 150)
fmodels <- Mods(linear = NULL, emax = 25,
logistic = c(50, 10.88111), exponential = 85,
betaMod = rbind(c(0.33, 2.31), c(1.39, 1.39)),
linInt = rbind(c(0, 1, 1, 1, 1),
c(0, 0, 1, 1, 0.8)),
doses=doses, placEff = 0, maxEff = 0.4,
addArgs=list(scal=200))
## Calculate doses giving an improvement of 0.3 over placebo
TD(fmodels, Delta=0.3)
## discrete version
TD(fmodels, Delta=0.3, TDtype ="discrete", doses=doses)
## doses giving 50% of the maximum effect
ED(fmodels, p=0.5)
ED(fmodels, p=0.5, EDtype = "discrete", doses=doses)
plot(fmodels, plotTD = TRUE, Delta = 0.3)
```

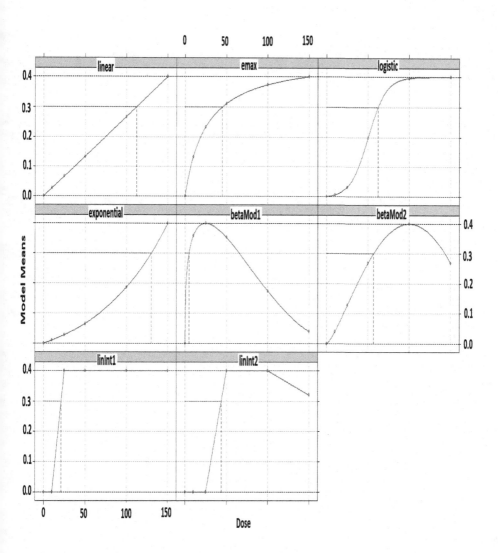

FIGURE 5.5: Dose determination by different model.

Part II

Bayesian in Time-to-Event Data Analysis

Chapter 6

Survival Analysis

Abstract

The survival analysis is widely adopted statistical analysis in oncology. Commonly, the Kaplan-Meier estimate and Cox proportional hazard models are performed in survival analysis. The Kaplan-Meier showed by assuming the censoring mechanism is non-informative. However, it gets violated some times. The informative censoring procedure using a Bayesian framework is suitable to overcome this violation. This chapter is dedicated to Bayesian survival analysis. Real-life data analysis is illustrated with OpenBUGS software. Similarly, survival analysis with R by Kaplan-Meier method, Cox PH model, Schoenfeld Residuals and other tools are theoretically explained.

6.1 Introduction

The objective of the survival analysis is to estimate and interpret hazard functions from survival data. Secondly, compare the hazard functions. Thirdly, explore the relationship of explanatory variables to survival time. Hazard function created from several groups.

Survival analysis comes with an analytical problem as censoring. Censoring comes while we have some information about individual survival time, but we do not have actual survival time.

The censoring data occurred if the event may not occur before the study end, the person is lost to follow-up during the study ends, and a person withdraws from the study due to other causes of death.

If the real survival time is equal to or greater than the observed survival time then it is defined as Right censoring.

Similarly, if the real survival time is less than or equal to the observed survival time, then it is defined as Left censoring.

Conventionally, the survival analysis is performed with hazard function. The hazard function $h(t)$ is defined as the instantaneous potential per unit time for the event to occur, given that the individual has survived up to time t.

6.1.1   Kaplan-Meier estimator

The survival data having censored data can be estimated by Kaplan-Meier estimator. It is a nonparametric estimator. The survival curves are compared by the Kaplan-Meier estimator. It is obtained as a product limit formula. The Kaplan-Meier estimator for the survival distribution function is estimated as

$$\hat{S}(t) = \prod_{t_j \leq t} (1 - \frac{d_j}{r_j}) \tag{6.1}$$

d_j is the person died till time t_j.

Now r_j is the persons at risk before time t_j. The variance of the Kaplan-Meier estimator is obtained as

$$\hat{\sigma}^2(t) = \hat{S}(t)^2 \sum_{t_j \leq t} \frac{d_j}{r_j(r_j - d_j)} \tag{6.2}$$

In absence of censoring, the term $\hat{S}(t)[1 - \hat{S}(t)]/n$ becomes to standard binomial variance estimator. The function to obtain Kaplan-Meier estimates in R is given below. The package "survival" is used to obtain the estimates.

```
Kaplan-Meier Using R

library("survival")
data(lung)
KM.result<-survfit(Surv(time, status) ~ 1, data=lung)
KM.result
```

```
Call: survfit(formula = Surv(time, status) ~ 1, data = lung)

      n  events  median 0.95LCL 0.95UCL
    228     165     310     285     363
```

```
Kaplan-Meier Plot R

library("survival")
library("ranger")
library("ggplot2")
library("dplyr")
library("ggfortify")
autoplot("KM.result")
```

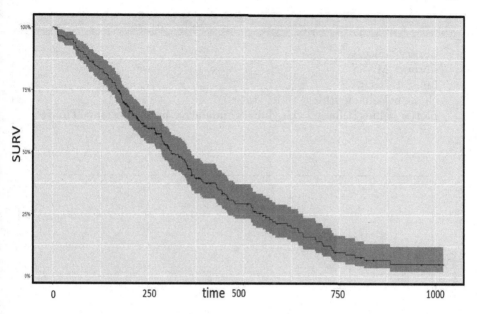

FIGURE 6.1: Kaplan-Meier plot R.

6.1.2 Nelson-Aalen estimator

Nelson-Aalen estimator is a nonparametric estimator. It is used to estimate the cumulative hazard rate function from censored survival data. Here, no distributional assumptions are required. It is more appropriate for data exploration through graphically. It is also known as: (1) Altshuler estimator, (2) Empirical cumulative hazard estimator, (3) Aalen-Nelson estimator. The Nelson-Aalen estimator for the cumulaive hazard rate function takes the form

$$\hat{A} = \sum_{t_j \leq t} \frac{d_j}{r_j} \tag{6.3}$$

Here, r_j is the number of individual at risk (not censored and alive). d_j is the person died till time t_j. This estimator is a increasing right-continous step function with increments of $\frac{d_j}{r_j}$ at the observed faliure times.

Nelson-Aalen estimator performs better when the sample size is small. It is asymptotically equivalent to Product Limit estimator and is also the nonparametric maximum likelihood estimator. It is commonly used to check the parametric model assumption and get a crude estimation of the hazard function.

```
Nelson-Aalen Estimator Plot Using R

library("mice")
library("MASS")
lung$status <- 2
ch <- nelsonaalen(lung, time, status)
plot(x = lung$time y = ch,ylab='Cumulative hazard', xlab='Time')
```

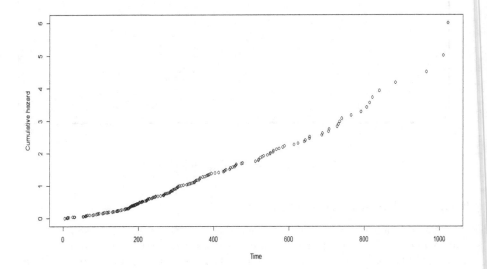

FIGURE 6.2: Nelson-Aalen estimator plot obtained by R.

6.2 Bayesian in Survival Analysis

Bayesian statistics comes as an alternative to the conventional approach. It helps to design and to analyze oncology data. Time-to-event outcomes are common in oncology research. Several complex issues in a time-to-event outcome can be handled with the Bayesian approach. In this chapter, we will show the Bayesian extension of survival in simple formation.

6.2.1 Cox's proportional hazards model

The Cox model specifies the hazard for individual i as

$$h_i(t) = h_0(t)e^{X_i(t)\beta} \tag{6.4}$$

where h_0 is an unspecified positive function of time called the baseline hazard, and β is a $p \times 1$ column vector of coefficients. The covaraites is defined by $X_i(t)$.

6.2.2 Hazard ratio

The hazard ratio for two subjects with fixed covariate vectors X_i and X_j are

$$\frac{h_i(t)}{h_j(t)} = \frac{h_0(t)e^{X_i\beta}}{h_0(t)e^{X_j\beta}} = \frac{e^{X_i\beta}}{e^{X_j\beta}} \qquad (6.5)$$

The term

$$\frac{h_i(t)}{h_j(t)}$$

is constant over time and the model is known as the proportional hazards model.

6.2.3 Partial likelihood function

Partial likelihood function is

$$PL(\beta) = \prod_{i=1}^{n}\prod_{t\geq 0}\{\frac{Y_i(t)r_i(\beta,t)}{\sum_j Y_j(t)r_j(\beta,t)}\}^{dN_i(t)} \qquad (6.6)$$

The log partial likelihood is presented as

$$l(\beta) = \sum_{i=1}^{n}\int_0^{\infty}[Y_i(t)X_i(t)\beta - log(\sum_j Y_j(t)r_j(t))]dN_i(t) \qquad (6.7)$$

The log partial likelihood with respect to β gives the $p \times 1$ score vector, $U(\beta)$:

$$U(\beta) = \sum_{i=1}^{n}\int_0^{\infty}[X_i(s) - \bar{x}(\beta,s)]dN_i(s) \qquad (6.8)$$

and

$$\bar{x}(\beta,s) = \frac{\sum Y_i(s)r_i(S)X_i(s)}{\sum Y_i(s)r_i(s)} \qquad (6.9)$$

with $Y_i(s)r_i(s)$ as the weights. The maximum partial likelihood estimator is found by solving the partial likelihood equation:

$$U(\hat{\beta}) = 0 \qquad (6.10)$$

Now $\hat{\beta}$ is consistent and asymptotically normally distributed with mean β with variance $\{EI(\beta)\}^{-1}$

Cox PH using R

```
library("survival")
data(lung)
a<-coxph(Surv(time, status) ~ ph.ecog,data=lung)
summary(a)
```

```
#R Output

coxph(formula = Surv(time, status) ~ ph.ecog, data = lung)

  n= 227, number of events= 164
   (1 observation deleted due to missingness)

          coef exp(coef) se(coef)      z Pr(>|z|)
ph.ecog 0.4759    1.6095   0.1134 4.198 2.69e-05 ***
---
Signif. codes:0 '***' 0.001 '**'0.01'*'0.05'.'0.1' '1

          exp(coef) exp(-coef) lower .95 upper .95
ph.ecog       1.61     0.6213     1.289      2.01

Concordance= 0.604  (se = 0.024 )
Likelihood ratio test= 17.57  on 1 df,    p=3e-05
Wald test            = 17.62  on 1 df,    p=3e-05
Score (logrank) test = 17.89  on 1 df,    p=2e-05
```

6.2.4   Stratified Cox model

Let that subjects $i = 1, ..., n_1$ are in stratum 1, subjects $n_{l+1}, ..., n_l + n_2$ are in stratum 2, and so on. The hazard for an individual i, who belongs to stratum k is

$$\lambda_k(t)e^{X_i\beta} \tag{6.11}$$

The overall loglikelihood

$$l(\beta) = \sum_{k=1} l_k(\beta) \tag{6.12}$$

The score vector and information matrix are $U(\beta) = \sum U_k(\beta)$ and $I(\beta) = \sum I_k(\beta)$ respectively.

```
Stratified Cox Model Using R

library("survival")
data(lung)
b<-coxph(Surv(time, status) ~ sex + strata(ph.ecog),data=lung)
summary(b)
```

```
#R Output

coxph(formula = Surv(time, status) ~ sex + strata(ph.ecog),
 data = lung)

 n= 227, number of events= 164
   (1 observation deleted due to missingness)

          coef exp(coef) se(coef)      z Pr(>|z|)
sex -0.5544    0.5744   0.1706  -3.25  0.00115 **
---
Signif. codes:0 '***' 0.001 '**' 0.01 '*' 0.05 '.' 0.1 ' ' 1

         exp(coef) exp(-coef) lower .95 upper .95
sex        0.5744      1.741     0.4112    0.8025

Concordance= 0.585  (se = 0.022 )
Likelihood ratio test= 11.09  on 1 df,    p=9e-04
Wald test              = 10.56  on 1 df,    p=0.001
Score (logrank) test = 10.81  on 1 df,    p=0.001
```

6.2.5 Wald-score and likelihood ratio tests

The Wald-score and likelihood ratio are useful for the Cox partial likelihood to test hypotheses about β. The likelihood ratio test is $2(l(\hat{\beta}) - l(\beta^{(0)}))$, twice the difference in the log partial likelihood at the initial and final estimates of $\hat{\beta}$.
The Wald test is $(\hat{\beta} - \beta^{(0)})'\hat{I}(\hat{\beta} - \beta^{(0)})$, where $\hat{I} = I(\hat{\beta})$ is the estimated information matrix at the solution.
The efficient score test statistic $U'(\beta^{(0)})I(\beta^{(0)})^{-1}U(\beta^{(0)})$ can be computed using only the first iteration of the Newton-Raphson algorithm.

6.2.6 Diagnostics for Cox's PH model

A large number of diagnostic methods for checking have been proposed over the year for Cox' proportional hazard (PGH) regression model, nut they are still not used as widely as they should be. The PH model [Cox (1972)] specifies

$$h(t; x) = h_0(t)e^{\beta' x} \qquad (6.13)$$

for the hazard function for the failure time T associated with a p-dimensional vector of covariates x, given an unknown underlying hazard function h_0 and a vector of coefficients β which must be estimated. The hazard function of the PH model is defined as,

$$S(t; x) = exp\{-\Delta_0(t)e^{\beta' x}\} \tag{6.14}$$

The cumulative hazard function Δ_0 corresponding to h_0.

$$In\{-InS(t; x)\} = In\Delta_0 + \beta' x \tag{6.15}$$

of the PH model is defined as,

$$S(t; x) = exp\{-\Delta_0(t)e^{\beta' x}\} \tag{6.16}$$

Any survival function $S(t; x)$ plotted on the complementary log-log scale, differs from $In\Delta_0$ by the constant amount $\beta' x$ throughout its duration.

Hence there are two functions. $S(t; x_1)$ and $S(t; x_2)$ for different values of the covariate vector x, will be parallel.

This gives the basic means of inspecting the PH assumption. Reliable estimates of $\hat{S}$ is important to take decision about plot.

A large amount of data available for each chosen x is significant to make a decision about the plot.

Diagnostics for Cox's PH Model Using R

```
library("survival")
data(lung)
res.cox<-coxph(Surv(time, status) ~ sex,data=lung)
res.cox
test.ph <- cox.zph(res.cox)
test.ph
```

#R Output

```
     chisq df      p
sex   2.86  1 0.091
GLOBAL 2.86  1 0.091
```

6.2.7   Schoenfeld residuals

Residuals from a fitted model are most easily understood when they express in some way the difference between observed data values and the corresponding fitted (predicted) values.

Large amount of data available for each chosen x is very important to take decision about plot. At the time i, of death or failure of unit or individual i, there is a risk set R_i; consisting of the individuals who have not yet failed (or been censored) so were at risk of failure at this time. The conditional probability that i failed, given that there was a failure at t_l is given by

$$p_i = \frac{h_i(t_i)}{\sum_{j\epsilon R_i} h_j(t_i)} = \frac{e^{\beta' x}}{\sum_{j\epsilon R_i} e^{\beta' x_j}} \tag{6.17}$$

The expected value $E(X|R_i)$ is

$$E(X|R_i) = \sum_{k\epsilon R_i} x_k p_k = \frac{\sum_{k\epsilon R_i} x_k e^{\beta' x_k}}{\sum_{j\epsilon R_i} e^{\beta' x_j}} \tag{6.18}$$

The vector is defined as

$$r_i = x_i - E(X|R_i) \tag{6.19}$$

The estimate of schoenfeld residual is

$$\hat{r}_i = x_i - \hat{E}(X|R_i) \tag{6.20}$$

The Schoenfeld residual is closely related to the estimation procedure of Cox's PH model.

Graphical Test for Proportional Hazards Using R

```
library("survival")
fit    <-    coxph(Surv(time,status)    ~    sex+factor(ph.ecog)+age,
data=lung,x=TRUE)
plot(cox.zph(fit))
```

6.3   Bayesian Survival Analysis Using R

Bayesian Survival Analysis Using R

```
library("survival")
library("BMA")
data(veteran)
veteran[1:10,]
test.bic.surv<- bic.surv(Surv(time,status) ~ ., data = veteran,
factor.type = TRUE)
summary(test.bic.surv, conditional=FALSE, digits=2)
plot(test.bic.surv)
imageplot.bma(test.bic.surv)
```

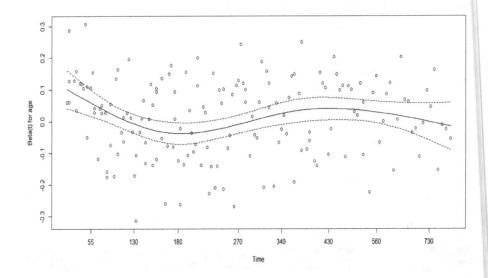

FIGURE 6.3: Beta(t) for age is obtained by imageplot.bme.

```
#R Script to Show Data

    trt celltype time status karno diagtime age prior
1    1 squamous    72      1    60        7  69     0
2    1 squamous   411      1    70        5  64    10
3    1 squamous   228      1    60        3  38     0
4    1 squamous   126      1    60        9  63    10
5    1 squamous   118      1    70       11  65    10
6    1 squamous    10      1    20        5  49     0
7    1 squamous    82      1    40       10  69    10
8    1 squamous   110      1    80       29  68     0
9    1 squamous   314      1    50       18  43     0
10   1 squamous   100      0    70        6  70     0
```

```
#R Output
```

```
bic.surv.formula(f = Surv(time, status) ~ ., data = veteran,
factor.type = TRUE)
  6  models were selected
 Best  5  models (cumulative posterior probability =  0.95 ):
                  p!=0       EV        SD      model 1  model 2
trt              11.3     0.02909    0.1058      .        .
celltype         84.6
        .smallcell         0.61564   0.3538    0.7121     .
        .adeno             0.97619   0.4965    1.1508     .
        .large             0.28260   0.2830    0.3251     .
karno           100.0    -0.03135   0.0052   -0.0309    -0.03
diagtime          5.4     0.00018   0.0020      .        .
age               6.1    -0.00036   0.0026      .        .
prior             5.6     0.00058   0.0054      .        .
nVar                                             2        1
BIC                                          -39.3626  -36.77
post prob                                      0.562     0.15
                  p!=0       EV        SD      model 3
trt              11.3     0.02909    0.1058    0.2573
celltype         84.6
        .smallcell         0.61564   0.3538    0.8196
        .adeno             0.97619   0.4965    1.1477
        .large             0.28260   0.2830    0.3930
karno           100.0    -0.03135   0.0052   -0.0311
diagtime          5.4     0.00018   0.0020      .
age               6.1    -0.00036   0.0026      .
prior             5.6     0.00058   0.0054      .
nVar                                             3
BIC                                          -36.1558
post prob                                      0.113
                 model 4    model 5
trt                .          .
celltype
        .smallcell       0.7208     0.7264
        .adeno           1.1643     1.1765
        .large           0.3215     0.3276
karno              -0.0318    -0.0311
diagtime            .          .
age                -0.0059      .
prior               .        0.0103
nVar                 3          3
BIC             -34.9292   -34.7553
post prob         0.061      0.056
```

6.3.1   BayesSurvival

> **PlotBayesSurv to Create Posterior Mean with Credible Band for the Survival Function or Cumulative Hazard.**
>
> ```
> library("BayesSurvival")
> library("simsurv")
> library("ggplot2")
> hazard.true <- function(t,x, betas, ...)
> 1.2×(5×(t+0.05)³-10 × (t+0.05)²+5×(t+0.05))+0.7
> sim.df <- data.frame(id = 1:1000)
> df <- simsurv(x = sim.df, maxt = 1, hazard = hazard.true)
> bs <- BayesSurv(df, "eventtime", "status")
> PlotBayesSurv(bs, object = "survival")
> cumhaz.plot + labs(title = "Cumulative hazard")
> ```

6.3.2   muhaz

> **Cumulative Hazard Plot with R**
>
> ```
> library("muhaz")
> library("survival")
> data(lung)
> attach(lung)
> fit <- pehaz(time,status)
> plot(fit)
> fit <- muhaz(time,status)
> summary(fit)
> plot(fit)
> ```

6.3.3   Bayesian in Kaplan-meier estimator

The Kaplan-Meier estimator stands as a product-limit method. The posterior distribution of the parameter is estimated through the Bayesian approach. It is estimated as the probability for the various ordered of censoring and recurrence time. It is the binomial distribution, for the ith ordered distribution by

$$d[i] \sim \text{binomoial}(q[i[, R[i])$$

(6.21)

Now $q[i]$ represent the probability of recurrence and $R[i]$ as the number at risk at the beginning of the ith ordered time. A beta prior for the $q[i]$ is suitable to estimate as

$$q[i] \sim \text{beta}(0.01, 0.01) \tag{6.22}$$

It used to estimate the posterior distribution for the recurrence probability. Now the recurrence probability is estimated as

$$P[T > t_{(i)} | T \geq t_{(i)}] \text{for i=1,2, .,m} \tag{6.23}$$

The number of ordered time/censored time is represented by m. Now at time point i, the number of persons at risk is defined as

$$r[i] = r[i-1] - c[i-1] - d[i-1] \tag{6.24}$$

for $i = 2, 3, ., m$, where m is the number of distinct ordered times. Like death, the censored can also be defined as

$$c[i] \sim \text{binomial}(qc[i], R[i]) \tag{6.25}$$

and

$$qc[i] \sim \text{beta}(0.01, 0.01) \tag{6.26}$$

Now distribution assumptions about death and censoring jointly specify the number at risk. Now the task is to generate the posterior distribution of $S(t_{(i)})$ as the conditional probabilities

$$P[T > t_{(i)} | T \geq t_{(i)}] \tag{6.27}$$

to obtain the Kaplan-Meier estimate. Suppose patients treated with "weekly cisplatin chemotherapy" is defined as arm=0 and "3-weekly cisplatin chemotherapy" as arm=1. The given below OpenBUGS code is useful to obtain the Kaplan-Meier as

---

Bayesian Kaplan-Meier with OpenBUGS

```
model;
{
for (i  in 1:m1){ d1[i] ~ dbin(q1[i],r1[i])}
for (i  in 1:m1){ ce1[i] ~ dbin(qc1[i],r1[i])}
for (i  in 1:m1){ q1[i] ~ dbeta (.01,.01)}
for (i  in 1:m1){ qc1[i] ~ dbeta (.01,.01)}
for(i  in 1:m1){ p[i]<-(r[i]-d[i])/r[i]}
for (i  in 1:m1){ p1[i]<-1-q1[i]}
r1[1]<- 35
for(i  in 2:m1){ r1[i]<-r1[i-1]-d1[i-1]-ce1[i-1]}
for (i  in 2:m1){ s1[i]<-s1[i-1]× p1[i]}
s1[1]<-p1[1]
for (i  in 1:m2){ d2[i]~ dbin(q2[i],r2[i])}
for (i  in 1:m2){ ce2[i]~ dbin(qc2[i],r2[i])}
for (i  in 1:m2){ q2[i]~ dbeta (.01,.01)}
for (i  in 1:m2){ qc2[i]~ dbeta (.01,.01)}
for(i  in 1:m2){ p2[i]<-(r2[i]-d2[i])/r2[i]}
for (i  in 1:m2){ p2[i]<-1-q2[i]}
r2[1]<- 19
for(i  in 2:m2){ r2[i]<-r2[i-1]-d2[i-1]-ce2[i-1]}
for (i  in 2:m2){ s2[i]<-s2[i-1] × p2[i]}
s2[1]<-p2[1]
}
#call the data #
list(m1 = 9,d1 = c(3,2,1,1,2,1,1,1,1),ce1 = c(1,1,2,0,3,0,5,6,4),
m2 = 10,d2 = c(2,2,1,2,2,4,2,2,1,1),
ce2 = c(0,0,0,0,0,0,0,0,0,0))
#Define the initial data#
list(q1 = c(.5,.5,.5,.5,.5,.5,.5,.5,.5),
q2 = c(.5,.5,.5,.5,.5,.5,.5,.5,.5,.5))
```

Now we performed the analysis with 20,000 observations as simulation. A burn-in of 1,000 and a refresh of 100 is considered. The conditional distribution for both the arm is presented below. The recurrence probability is defined as

$$S[i] = S(t_{(i)}) \qquad (6.28)$$

Similarly, the conditional probabilty is defined as

$$P[i] = P[T > t_{(i)} | T \geq t_{(i)}] \qquad (6.29)$$

The link between condition probability and recurrence probability is

$$S[i] = S[i-1]P[i] \qquad (6.30)$$

The curve between $\hat{S}_1(t)$ and $\hat{S}_2(t)$ are useful for survival comparison between the arms.

TABLE 6.1: Posterior estimates survival estimates for Arm=1

Parameter	Mean	SD	val2.5pc	median	val97.5pc
s1[1]	0.91	0.04	0.80	0.92	0.98
s1[2]	0.85	0.05	0.72	0.86	0.94
s1[3]	0.82	0.06	0.68	0.82	0.93
s1[4]	0.79	0.06	0.64	0.79	0.90
s1[5]	0.72	0.07	0.56	0.72	0.86
s1[6]	0.68	0.08	0.51	0.69	0.83
s1[7]	0.64	0.08	0.47	0.65	0.80
s1[8]	0.59	0.09	0.40	0.59	0.76
s1[9]	0.47	0.12	0.22	0.48	0.69
p1[1]	0.91	0.04	0.80	0.92	0.98
p1[2]	0.93	0.04	0.83	0.94	0.99
p1[3]	0.96	0.03	0.87	0.97	0.99
p1[4]	0.96	0.03	0.86	0.97	0.99
p1[5]	0.91	0.05	0.77	0.92	0.98
p1[6]	0.94	0.05	0.81	0.96	0.99
p1[7]	0.94	0.05	0.80	0.95	0.99
p1[8]	0.91	0.07	0.71	0.93	0.99
p1[9]	0.79	0.16	0.39	0.83	0.99

6.3.4 Bayesian Cox proportional hazards model

The Cox proportional hazards model is defined as

$$h(t, X) = h_0(t)\exp(\sum_{i=1}^{i=p} \beta_i X_i) \tag{6.31}$$

The regression parameter is defined as X_i. Similarly, the baseline hazard function is $h_0(t)$. Now covariate is defined as X_i. The baseline hazard function is presented with time, but the covariates are not the functions of t. Further, at the time t the hazard function is presented as

$$h(t) = \frac{\lim_{\Delta t \to \infty} P(t \leq T < t + \Delta t | T \geq t)}{\Delta t} \tag{6.32}$$

Now the hazard function can be defined with $S(t)$ to obtain the Bayesian inference

$$h(t) = \frac{[dS(t)/dt]}{S(t)} \tag{6.33}$$

The survival function is

$$S(t) = P(T > t) \tag{6.34}$$

The hazard ratio is presented as

$$\text{HR} = \frac{h(t, X^*)}{h(t, X)} \tag{6.35}$$

TABLE 6.2: Posterior estimates survival estimates for Arm=2

Parameter	Mean	SD	val2.5pc	median	val97.5pc
s2[1]	0.89	0.06	0.72	0.90	0.98
s2[2]	0.78	0.09	0.58	0.79	0.93
s2[3]	0.73	0.09	0.52	0.74	0.89
s2[4]	0.63	0.10	0.40	0.63	0.82
s2[5]	0.52	0.11	0.30	0.52	0.74
s2[6]	0.31	0.10	0.13	0.30	0.53
s2[7]	0.20	0.09	0.06	0.19	0.41
s2[8]	0.10	0.06	0.01	0.091	0.27
s2[9]	0.05	0.04	0.00	0.037	0.18
s2[10]	0.00	0.00	0	0	0.00
p2[1]	0.89	0.06	0.72	0.90	0.98
p2[2]	0.88	0.07	0.69	0.89	0.98
p2[3]	0.93	0.06	0.76	0.95	0.99
p2[4]	0.85	0.09	0.63	0.87	0.98
p2[5]	0.83	0.10	0.58	0.85	0.97
p2[6]	0.59	0.14	0.29	0.60	0.86
p2[7]	0.66	0.17	0.28	0.68	0.94
p2[8]	0.50	0.22	0.09	0.50	0.90
p2[9]	0.50	0.28	0.02	0.50	0.97
p2[10]	0.01	0.07	0.00	0	0.08

Now the same covariate X can be separated as X^* and X. The term X^* shows the one category of a variable X. Similarly, X defined another category. The HR is defined as

$$\text{HR} = \exp(\sum_{i=1}^{i=p} \beta_i(X_i^* - X_i)) \tag{6.36}$$

Now the Bayesian specify the prior distribution of β. It used to obtain the hazard ratio. If $X = 0$ and $X^* = 1$ then hazard ratio formed as

$$HR(\beta) = \exp(\beta) \tag{6.37}$$

The OpenBUGS codes is provided to compute the hazard ratio through Bayesian approach.

TABLE 6.3: Posterior estimates Hazard Ratio for Arm=2 with respect to Arm=1

Parameter	Mean	SD	val2.5pc	median	val97.5pc
HR	4.763	2.645	1.375	4.022	11.52

Bayesian Cox PH with OpenBUGS

```
model
{
for(i in 1:N) {
for(j in 1:T) {
Y[i,j] <- step(obs.t[i]-t[j]+eps)
dN[i, j] <- Y[i, j] × step(t[j + 1]-obs.t[i]-eps) × fail[i]
}}
for(j in 1:T) {
for(i in 1:N) {
dN[i, j] ~ dpois(Idt[i, j])
Idt[i, j] <- Y[i, j] × exp(beta × x1[i]) × dL0[j]
}
dL0[j] ~ dgamma(mu[j], c)
mu[j] <- dL0.star[j] × c
S.treat[j] <- pow(exp(-sum(dL0[1 : j]))
exp(beta × -0.5))
S.placebo[j] <- pow(exp(-sum(dL0[1 : j]))
exp(beta × 0.5))
}
c <- 0.001
r <- 0.1
for (j in 1 : T) {
dL0.star[j] <- r × (t[j + 1]-t[j])
}
beta ~ dnorm(0.0,0.000001)
HR<-exp(beta)
}
list(N = 44,T = 16,eps=1.0E-20,obs.t = c(1, 1, 2, 2, 3, 4, 4, 5, 5,
8, 8, 8, 8, 11,11,12,12,12,15,15,17,22,23,6,6, 6, 6, 7, 9, 10,
10,11,13,16,17,19,20,22,23,25,32,32,34,35),
fail=c(1,1,1,1,1,1,1,1,1,1,1,1,1,1,1,1,1,1,1,1,
1, 1, 1, 1, 1, 1,1,0, 1, 0, 1, 0, 0, 1, 1, 0,
0, 0, 1, 1, 0, 0, 0, 0, 0),
x1 = c(0.5, 0.5, 0.5, 0.5, 0.5, 0.5, 0.5, 0.5, 0.5, 0.5,
0.5, 0.5, 0.5, 0.5, 0.5, 0.5, 0.5, 0.5,0.5,0.5, 0.5, 0.5,
0.5, -0.5,-0.5, -0.5,-0.5, -0.5,-0.5,-0.5, -0.5,-0.5,-0.5,
-0.5,-0.5,-0.5,-0.5,-0.5,-0.5,-0.5,-0.5, -0.5, -0.5, -0.5),
t = c(1, 2, 3, 4, 5, 6, 7, 8, 10, 11, 12, 13, 15, 16,
17, 22, 23))
list(beta = 0.0,dL0 = c(1.0,1.0,1.0,1.0,1.0,1.0,1.0,1.0,
1.0,1.0,1.0,1.0,1.0,1.0,1.0, 1.0))
```

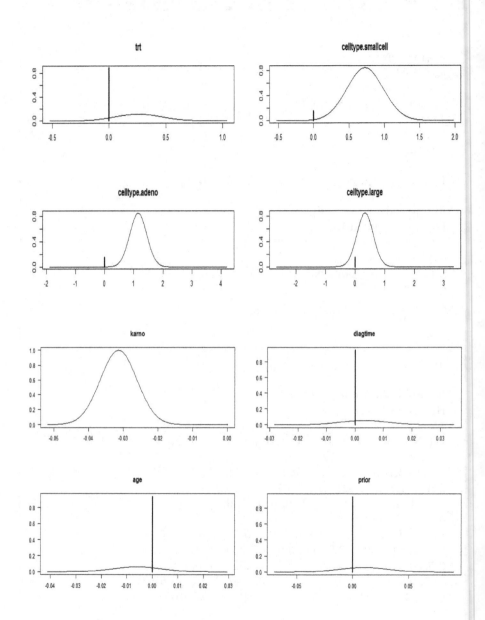

FIGURE 6.4: Posterior estimates convergence plot.

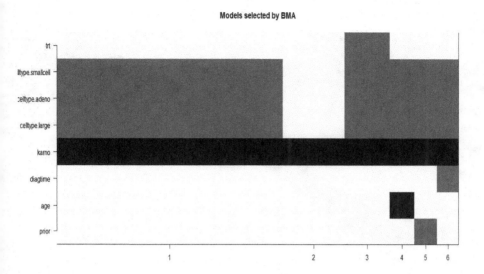

FIGURE 6.5: Bayesian model average.

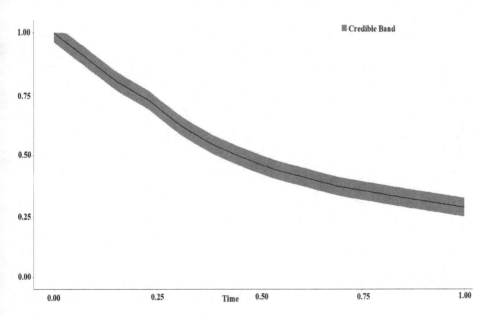

FIGURE 6.6: Posterior estimate plot of survival function.

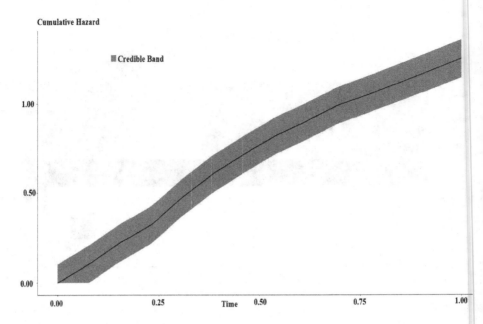

FIGURE 6.7: Posterior estimate plot of cumulative hazard.

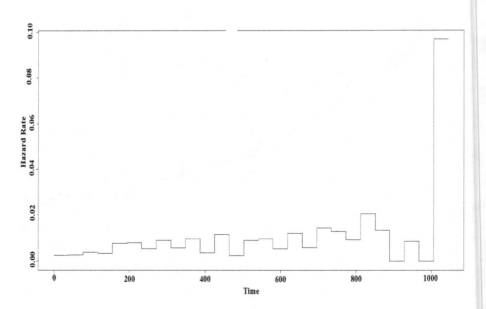

FIGURE 6.8: Estimates piecewise exponential hazard function.

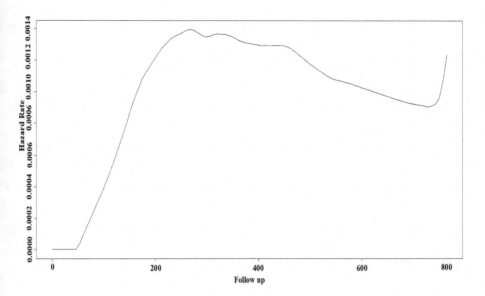

FIGURE 6.9: Posterior estimate plot of cumulative hazard.

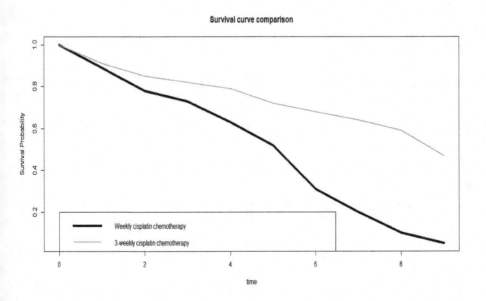

FIGURE 6.10: Survival curve comparison.

Chapter 7

Competing Risk Data Analysis

Abstract

Survival analysis data comes with multiple and mutually exclusive events. The application of competing risk modeling helps to account different causes of death. There are several techniques to work with competing risk modeling to prioritize the specific cause. Several techniques are available to work with the cause-specific framework, mixture models, sub-distribution hazard, and method of pseudo-observations. This chapter is dedicated toward different methodology to handle cause-specific model. Details review of competing risk model is available. Theory about competing Risk as Bivariate Random Variable, Cumulative Incidence Rate, and Cause-specific hazard model are discussed. The illustration to perform competing risk model with R and Open-BUGS are elaborated. This chapter will be helpful to perform a competing risk model in oncology or time-to-event data.

7.1   Introduction

The occurrence of Competing risk is prevalent in oncology. The reason for death for the treated cancer patients may be different, and it is defined as 'Competing Risk'. Now, the reason of death may be a local recurrence, distant metastases, occurrence of a secondary tumor. There are different strategies to deal with competing risks with survival analysis. The conventional survival suggests pursuing with cause-specific death modeling. It occurs when there are at least two possible ways that a person can fail, but only one such failure type can occur. The situation in which an individual can experience more than one type of event [14, 15].The failure to achieve independence between the time to an event and the censoring mechanism [16, 17].The concept of competing risks as the situation where one type of event 'either precludes the occurrence of another event under investigation or fundamentally alters the probability of occurrence of this other event [18].

Suppose, T is a continuous positive random variable provides survival time.

The probability density function (pdf) is defined as $f(t)$. The cumulative distribution function (cdf) is defined as

$$F(t) = Pr\{T \le t\} \tag{7.1}$$

Now the survival function of the probability of being alive at t. The survival function of the probability of being alive at t is presented as.

$$S(t) = Pr\{T > t\} \tag{7.2}$$

The hazard function is defined as

$$\lambda(t) = [\frac{f(t)}{S(t)}] \tag{7.3}$$

The cumulative hazard function is defined as

$$\Delta(t) = \int_0^t \lambda(\mu)d\mu \tag{7.4}$$

The survival function at time t is presented as

$$S(t) = exp\{-\Delta(t)\} \tag{7.5}$$

7.2   Competing Risk as Bivariate Random Variable

Let Censoring variable(C) and Time variable(T).Survival data are usually presented as a bivariate random variable or pair (C, T).If $C = 1$ then the first member of the pair is defined by T. The term T is time at which the event occurred.

If $C = 0$ then T is the time at which the observation was censored. Further, C can be extended into 0 and i.

Now $C = i, i = 1, ...p$ i represents the type of the first failure/event observed and T is the time at which the event of type i occurred. Now $C = 0$, If the observation is censored $C = i, i = 1, ...p$ otherwise.

For example, if $T = i, i = 1, ...p, i$ is the sepecific event and T_i is the duration of specific event. $T = i, i = 1, 2, 3, i = 1$, and T_1 is time to local relapse.

$i = 2$, and T_2 is time to distant relapse.

$i = 3$, and T_3 is time to death.

when $C = i$,then $T = min(T_1, T_2, T_3)$ otherwie $C = 0$.

7.3 Cumulative Incidence Rate

If it confirmed that if $C \neq 0$ then cumulative incidence function (CIF) required to present. Suppose the total number of observations are defined as N. However, if among the N observations some did not yet experience any of the p types of events, then censored observations are present in the dataset. The CIF for any event of type $i(i = 1, 2, ...p)$ is defined as the joint probability

$$F_i(t) = P(T \leq t, C = i) \qquad (7.6)$$

It is the probability that an event of any type occurs at or before time t. Hence,

$$F(t) = P(T \leq t) = \sum_{i=1}^{p} P(T \leq t, C = i) = \sum_{i=1}^{p} F_i(t) \qquad (7.7)$$

The probability that an event i does not occur by time t can be denoted as

$$S_i(t) = P(T > t, C = i) \qquad (7.8)$$

When the competing risks are not present the overall distribution function spans the interval $[0, 1]$.

7.4 Competing Risk Model Using R

A step-by-step procedure used to run R script to generate compting risk data, competing risk plot is detailed below.

```
Competing Risk Plot Using Timepoints

library("cmprsk")
library("survival")
os <- rexp(100)
death<-sample(1:2,100,replace=TRUE)
arm<- factor(sample(1:2,100,replace=TRUE), 1:2,c('arm1','arm2'))
competigndata<-cuminc(os,death,arm)
plot(competigndata,lty=1,color=1:4)
fit=cuminc(os,death)
fit
```

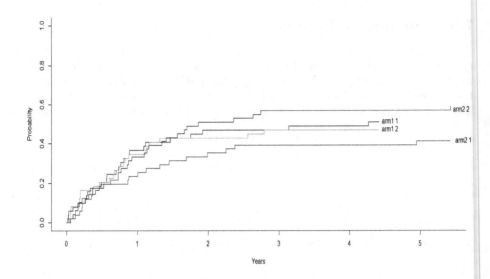

FIGURE 7.1: Armwise cumulative hazard comparison.

```
#R Output

Estimates and Variances:
$est
          1    2    3    4    5
1 1 0.30 0.41 0.43 0.44 0.46
1 2 0.34 0.47 0.52 0.52 0.53

$var
            1         2         3         4         5
1 1 0.002135 0.0024856 0.0025274 0.0025562 0.0026351
1 2 0.002282 0.0025567 0.0025940 0.0025940 0.0026136
```

```
#The CIF Estimates at 1,2,3 and 4 Yearss is Obtained by Function
Using Timepoints

timepoints(fit,times=c(1,2,3,4))
```

```
#R Output

$est
        1    2    3    4
1 1 0.30 0.41 0.43 0.44
1 2 0.34 0.47 0.52 0.52

$var
            1           2          3          4
1 1 0.00213530 0.002485680 0.002527465 0.002556282
1 2 0.00228206 0.002556745 0.002594095 0.002594095
```

7.5 Cause-Specific Hazard Model

Survival analysis data comes with multiple and mutually exclusive events. The application of competing risk modeling helps to account different causes of death. There are several techniques to work with competing risk modeling to prioritize the specific cause. There are several techniques to work cause-specific framework [14], mixture models [19], sub-distribution hazard [20], and method of pseudo-observations [21]. Details review of competing risk model is available [22]. Other techniques like machine learning through random forest method [23] are widely adopted in competing risk modeling [23, 24]. Suppose there are K coupled. The cumulative incidence functions $F_k(t)$. First-derivate can be presented as

$$\frac{dF_k(t)}{dt} = \left(1 - \sum_{k'=1}^{K} F_{k'}(t)\right) \lambda_k(t) \tag{7.9}$$

Now $\lambda_k(t)(\geq 0, \forall t > 0)$ shows that kth cause-specific hazard function. The equation can be reformulated as $\forall k$:

$$\sum_{k=1}^{K} \frac{dF_k(t)}{dt} = \left(1 - \sum_{k'=1}^{K} F_{k'}(t)\right) \sum_{k=1}^{K} \lambda_k(t) \tag{7.10}$$

$$\frac{dE(t)}{E(t)} = -\sum_{k} \lambda_k(t) \tag{7.11}$$

Now the event-free probability function is presented as $E(t)$,

$$E(t) = 1 - \sum_{k=1}^{K} F_k(t) \tag{7.12}$$

It can be obtained as

$$E(t) = \prod_{k=1}^{K} S_k(t) \tag{7.13}$$

If $S_k(t)$ stands with unadjusted survival function. let the causes are k. It is defined as

$$S_k(t) = \exp(-\int_{t'=0}^{t} \lambda_k(t')dt') \tag{7.14}$$

It can be obtained as

$$0 \leq S_k(t) \leq 1, \forall k = 1, ..., K, t \geq 0 \tag{7.15}$$

It is obtained as $S_k(0) = 1$. The one-dimensional integration can be obtained as

$$F_k(t) = \int_{t'=0}^{t} (\prod_{k'=1}^{K} S_k(t'))\lambda_k(t')dt' \tag{7.16}$$

It can be reformed as Weibull survival model as

$$\lambda_k(t) = \alpha_k \gamma_k t^{\alpha_k - 1} \tag{7.17}$$

$$S_k(t) = \exp(-\gamma_k t^{\alpha_k}) \tag{7.18}$$

It leads to cumulative incidence functions(CIF) with two competing risks ($K = 2$).

$$F_1(t) = -\alpha_1 \gamma_1 \int_0^t \mu^{\alpha_1 - 1} e^{\gamma_1 \mu^{\alpha_1} + \mu^{\alpha_2}} \tag{7.19}$$

Bayesian inference with Markov chain Monte Carlo (MCMC) useful to obtain the inference.

7.6   Bayesian Information Criteria

Different models can be formulated and thereafter models can be compared with Bayesian information criterion (BIC) [25]. It is an evaluation criterion in terms of the posterior probability [26]. Suppose there are $M_1, M_2, ..., M_r$ types of model and assigned as r candidate models. Let the parametric distribution is defined as $f_i(x|\theta_i)(\theta_i \in \Theta_i \in R^{k_i})$ The prior distribution $\pi_i(\theta_i)$ Let $M_1, M_2, ..., M_r$ be r candidate models, and assume that each model of the k_i-dimensional parameter vector θ_i. Now the number of observations are $x_n = \{x_1, ..., x_n\}$. The probability of x_n is defined as

$$p_i(x_n) = \int f_i(x_n|\theta_i)\pi_i(\theta_i)d\theta_i \tag{7.20}$$

The posterior probability of the ith can be defined as $P(M_i)$.

$$P(M_i|x_n) = \frac{p_j(x_n)P(M_j)}{\sum_{j=1}^{r} p_j(x_n)P(M_j)}, i = 1, 2, ..., r \tag{7.21}$$

Posterior probability represents ith model when x_n are observed. The model is selected from r models. The process is to consider the model that comes with the highest probability. The model maximize the numerator $p_i(x_n)P(M_i)$ is defined as best model.

It is assumed that the prior probability $P(M_i)$ are similar in all the models. It maximizes the marginal likelihood through $p_i(x_n)$ among the data selected.

$$\frac{P(M_1|x_n)}{P(M_2|x_n)} = \frac{p_1(x_n)}{p_2(x_n)} \frac{P(M_1)}{P(M_2)} \tag{7.22}$$

The Bayes factor is defined as

$$B_{12} = \frac{p_1(x_n)}{p_2(x_n)} = \frac{f_1(x_n|\theta_1)\pi_1(\theta_1)d\theta_1}{f_1(x_n|\theta_1)\pi_2(\theta_2)d\theta_2} \tag{7.23}$$

Fine and Gray Test Using R

```
data("mgus2")
head(mgus2)
etime <- with(mgus2, ifelse(pstat==0, futime, ptime))
event <- with(mgus2, ifelse(pstat==0, 2× death, 1))
event <- factor(event, 0:2, labels=c('censor', 'pcm', 'death'))
pdata <- finegray(Surv(etime, event) ~ ., data=mgus2)
fgfit <- coxph(Surv(fgstart, fgstop, fgstatus) ~ age,weight=fgwt,
data=pdata)
summary(fgfit)
```

#R Output

```
Call:
coxph(formula = Surv(fgstart, fgstop, fgstatus) ~ age,
data = pdata,weights = fgwt)

  n= 41775, number of events= 115

        coef exp(coef)  se(coef)        z Pr(>|z|)
age -0.016617  0.983521  0.007008  -2.371   0.0177 *
---
Signif.codes: 0 '***' 0.001 '**' 0.01 '*' 0.05 '.' 0.1 ' ' 1
    exp(coef) exp(-coef) lower .95 upper .95
age    0.9835      1.017    0.9701    0.9971

Concordance= 0.539  (se = 0.024 )
Likelihood ratio test= 5.35  on 1 df,    p=0.02
Wald test           = 5.62  on 1 df,    p=0.02
Score (logrank) test = 5.63  on 1 df,    p=0.02
```

7.7   Illustration Using R

```
Illustration Using R

library("survival")
library("BMA")
os <- rexp(100)
death<-sample(1:2,100,replace=TRUE)
arm<-rbinom(100, 1,.5)
age<-rnorm(100,50,10)
diagtime<-rnorm(100,5,1)
cdata<-data.frame(os,death,arm,age,diagtime)
test.bic.surv<- bic.surv(Surv(os,death) ~., data =cdata)
summary(test.bic.surv, conditional=FALSE, digits=2)
imageplot.bma(test.bic.surv)
```

```
#R Output

Call:
bic.surv.formula(f = Surv(os, death) ~ .,
data = cdata)


  Six models were selected
Best  5  models (cumulative posterior probability=0.96):

          p!=0    EV       SD       model 1   model 2
arm       12.9   -0.0243  0.120       .         .
age       36.1   -0.0072  0.012       .       -0.019
diagtime  11.9    0.0101  0.065       .         .

nVar                                  0         1
BIC                                 0.000     1.179
post prob                           0.484     0.268


          p!=0    EV       SD       model 3   model 4   model 5
arm       12.9   -0.0243  0.120       .       -0.125    -0.269
age       36.1   -0.0072  0.012       .         .       -0.023
diagtime  11.9    0.0101  0.065     0.113       .         .

nVar                                  1         1         2
BIC                                 3.541     3.808     4.290
post prob                           0.082     0.072     0.057
```

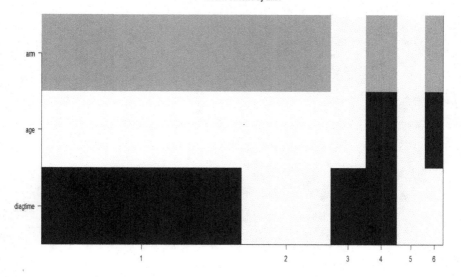

FIGURE 7.2: Comparison of Bayesian Moving average.

Chapter 8

Frailty Data Analysis

Abstract

Disease progression by recurrence, metastases are common in cancer. However, disease progression is dependent on individual-level effect. Several unknown factors are contributing to disease progression. Survival analysis of disease progression is useful. It makes it essential to accommodate several contributing factors on disease progression by frailty model. Frailty model is a branch of survival analysis.

This chapter is dedicated to frailty modelling. There are several techniques to work with frailty data to make survival analysis robust. Different methodology to handle frailty data analysis is presented. Data analysis with frailty model is prepared with R. Further, Bayesian inference of frailty modelling is presented. There are several techniques to work with frailty data to make survival analysis robust. This chapter is dedicated to different methodology to handle frailty data analysis. Details review of frailty data analysis is available. Theory about frailty data analysis is discussed. Example to handle frailty data analysis is illustrated with R. The Bayesian counterpart of Frailty data analysis also explained and presented by examples.

8.1 Introduction

A cancer patient may be observed with several events after or during the first treatment. For example, the patient opted for the head, and cancer may appear with disease recurrence or metastases disease. Cancer patients may experience recurrent even in the superficial tumor. The entire chance of recurrence is dependent on patient-level influence or can be defined as the individual-level effect. There could be several unknown factors that are contributing to disease appearance. The data handling technique on the recurrent event is conventionally known as survival analysis. However, the inclusion of several factors contribution at the individual level presents the extension of conventional survival model as a frailty model. One patient is defined as frail if he is having a higher/lower of exposure. Due to this, he is having a different disease relapse rate than others. Comprehensively, a different individual has different disease relapse rate. It introduces the term frailty. The frailty term is utilized as different individuals are at different risks even though it is assumed that they are at the same risk at treatment initiation. It becomes interesting while the appearance of other factors like age, sex, district are considered. Frailty term is used to serve as an unobservable random effect shared by subjects having similar risk in the analysis. Inclusion of random effect part help to describe the excess risk of mortality rate. A frailty data analysis is an extension of the survival model. The random effect component is attached to the conventional survival data model. However, conventional survival model always considered the random effect component. One extended random effect component is joined in the survival model and defined as a frailty model. The random effect can be utilized in the univariate data to make it more flexible. It becomes attractive in multivariate modeling. In oncology, multiple recurrent events may occur. The application of frailty model becomes attractive in case of multiple recurrent event modeling. Suppose the hazard function is defined as

$$Y\mu(t) \tag{8.1}$$

The term Y is unknown parameter and hazard function is $\mu(t)$. Y is useful toward random effect modeling. There are several unknown parameters, and those can be pushed as random components. It helps to make unknown values by integrating the random component. Now random effects may be reflected as the effect of unobserved covariates. Now the term K can be assumed as Poisson distribution with mean Yk. It can be conditioned with Y having parameter k. It can be formulated as Y with gamma distribution. It can be integrated out by the relevant time period. Survival data can not be avoided in oncology. It is the most common dataset. Medical oncology treated patients are followed for the primary outcome of a study as death or relapse. However, the censoring of the event is natural phenomena. Censoring becomes right while the time of interest is not measured, but the lower bound is observed. Handling right censoring data is different and challenging [27]. Widely used method for survival data is proportional hazard model. However, generated inference from the Cox proportional hazard model is applicable as identically independently distributed individuals. Perhaps, individuals may be exposed to different risk, even after maintaining other risk factors. Sometimes, patients may belong to different cluster or regions. It may be assumed that the individual belongs to the same cluster behave similarly. The intention of the multicentric clinical trial is about to prioritize the cluster-specific inference. The frailty model helps to account the heterogeneity at the baseline level. It is an extension of the proportional hazard model, while hazard function is dependent on unobservable random quantity. It is called as frailty. Distributional form of the frailty model can be assumed-the distribution of the frailties considered as gamma frailty. Gamma frailty model is widely used due to mathematical acceptability. The linear model is the extention of the generalized linear mixed effect model by lognormal frailty [28]. There are different multivariate formation by frailty data distribution [29]. The relation between baseline to time to event plays a crucial role. Different distribution formation is required to approach different frailty distribution [30]. Generally, the gamma distribution is a widely accepted choice for frailty distribution. The widely used R package is survival. Function available coxph() in survival package is useful to handle frailties as a semi-parametric model. Similarly, frailtypack package [31] provides the gamma frailty models as a semi-parametric estimation. The Weibull is the parametric choice. It can also be used in frailtypack package. The coxme [32] and phmm [33] functions also work in a similar direction with lognormal frailty model. But a large choice of parametric distributions is available in parfm [34], an R package. The gamma, inverse Gaussian, lognormal, Weibull, Gompertz, log-logistic are available in parfm. The parametric distributional estimation is performed by marginal log-likelihood maximization. Frailty distribution data is dependent with individual level variation.

8.2   Frailty Model

The frailty model is defined in terms of the conditional hazard Suppose the hazard function is assumed as

$$h_{ij}(t|u_i) = h_0(t)u_i\exp(x_{ij}^T\beta) \tag{8.2}$$

with $i \in I = \{1, ..., G\}$ and $j \in J_i = \{1, ..., n_i\}$. Now the $h_0(.)$ is considered as the baseline hazard function. The term u_i is assumed as frailty term for the covariates i, x_{ij}. The regression coefficient is defined as β. It is possible to obatain the univariate frailty model for n_i subjects [35]. Otherwise it is defindd as shared frailty model [28, 29]. Now the baseline hazard can be defined through the parametric approach. The term Ψ is formulated with the regression coefficient the parfm package available in Weibull, exponential, lognormal and log-logistic to serve the parametric distribution.

8.3   Motivating Example

Recently, a total of 50,381 patients data of multidisciplinary hepatocellular carcinoma (HCC) is analyzed through frailty modeling [36]. The type of hospital is considered in this illustration. The relation between the overall risk of death and type of hospital is figured through frailty. They used the multivariable Cox shared frailty modeling. Similarly, to explore the distance to

travel to get treatment among head and neck cancer patients are established
by Cox shared frailty model [37]. The overall survival(OS) was evaluated.

```
#Example1

      time cens   xcoord      ycoord     age sex wbc   tpi  district
  24   1    1    0.4123484 0.4233738 44   1  281.0 4.87  1
  62   3    1    0.3925028 0.4531422 72   1   0.0  7.10  1
  68   4    1    0.4167585 0.4520397 68   0   0.0  5.12  1
 128   9    1    0.4244763 0.4123484 61   1   0.0  2.90  1
 129   9    1    0.4145535 0.4520397 26   1   0.0  6.72  1
 163  15    1    0.4013230 0.4785006 67   1  27.9  1.50  1
```

```
# Output1

   Generalized accelerated failure time frailty model:
Call:
frailtyGAFT(formula = Surv(time, cens) ~ age + sex
  +wbc+tpi+baseline(age,sex,wbc,tpi)+frailtyprior("car",
     district), data = d, mcmc = mcmc, prior = prior,
Proximity = E)


Posterior means for regression coefficients:
            Mean    Median Std    95%HPD-Low  95%HPD-Upp
Intercept   8.58    8.60   0.28   7.98        9.14
age        -0.05   -0.05   0.00  -0.05       -0.04
sex        -0.26   -0.28   0.16  -0.53        0.06
wbc        -0.00   -0.00   0.00  -0.00       -0.00
tpi        -0.06   -0.06   0.01  -0.09       -0.02
Bayes factors for LDTFP covariate effects:
intercept  age    sex   wbc    tpi  overall  normality
 130.95    11.62  1.26  14.01  0.48 7.88      994.86
```

```
#Kidney Data Fit with Gamma Frailty Distribution

library("parfm")
head(kidney)
kidney$ sex <- kidney$sex - 1
mod <- parfm(Surv(time, status) ~ sex + age, cluster='id',
data=kidney, dist='exponential', frailty='gamma')
mod
ci.parfm(mod, level=0.05)['sex',]
u <- predict(mod)
plot(u, sort='i')
```

```
#R Output on Gamma Distribution Fit

   Frailty distribution: gamma
   Baseline hazard distribution: Exponential
   Loglikelihood: -333.248

          ESTIMATE SE    p-val
   theta   0.301   0.156
   lambda  0.025   0.014
   sex    -1.485   0.396 <.001 ***
   age     0.005   0.011 0.657
   ---
Signif.codes:0 '***' 0.001 '**' 0.01'*' 0.05 '.' 0.1 ' '1

   Kendall's Tau: 0.131
```

```
# R Output Confidence Interval Fit

 low   up
 0.104 0.492
```

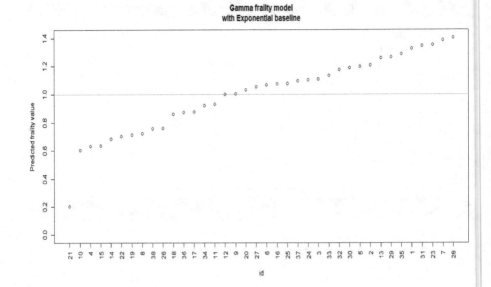

FIGURE 8.1: Gamma frailty model prediction.

```
#Kidney Data Fit with Different Distribution
```
```
kidney.parfm <- select.parfm(Surv(time, status) ~ sex + age,
cluster='id', data=kidney,dist=c('exponential','weibull','gompertz',
'loglogistic','lognormal'),frailty=c('gamma','ingau','possta'))
kidney.parfm
plot(kidney.parfm)
```

```
# R Output with Parametric Frailty Models

### - Parametric frailty models - ###
Progress status:
  'ok' = converged
  'nc' = not converged

                Frailty
Baseline         gamma   invGau   posSta
exponential.........ok......ok......ok....
Weibull.............ok......ok......ok....
Gompertz...........ok......nc......ok....
loglogistic........ok......ok......ok....
lognormal..........ok......ok......ok....
```

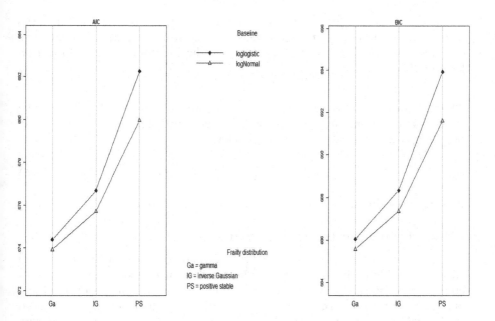

FIGURE 8.2: Estimates through different distribution.

8.4   Bayesian in Frailty Survival

The Bayesian counterpart of frailty survival model becomes interesting for researchers. Bayesian is applicable in different clinical; trial study design. Similarly, it is applicable to survival analysis. Bayesian works with prior distribution, design, monitoring, and data analysis. Perhaps, there is some limitation about the application of Bayesian toward prior distribution selection.

8.4.1   Frailty modeling

Frailty model can be adopted in any distribution if $Y \geq 0$. The univariate form is mentioned in equation 8.1. The parametric expression can be defined as $\mu(t)$. It helps to make the regression model with the Cox proportional model as

$$Y \exp(\beta' z)\mu_0(t) \tag{8.3}$$

The covariate is presented as z. The regression coefficient is β. If $z = 0$ then the hazard function becomes to $\mu_0(t)$. It is possible to make $\mu_0(t)$ as parametric or nonparametric. If covariate is absent then the conditional survival function becomes

$$S(t|Y) = \exp(-YM(t)) \tag{8.4}$$

The integrated conditional hazard is formulated as $M(t) = \int_0^t \mu(u)d\mu$. The term Y may become independent and not observed. In this context, it may be integrated out as expression given below.

$$S(t) = \int_0^\infty (-yM(T))g(y)dy \tag{8.5}$$

It is only possible while the frailty is continuous distribution.

8.4.2   Frailty on recurrent events

The frailty is assumed as a random effect for the subject. No individual effect is considered in this context. The conditional Poisson model is considered. It provides scope about any time point about the hazard of a subject about the appearance of a new event. The Poisson distribution is measured by $Y\mu(t)$. This model is defined as the time since the start of the process. Suppose the entire interval is 0 to t and the total number of events is K. The mean is $YM(t)$. The expression of probability term becomes

$$\Pr(K = k) = (-1)^k \{M(t)\}^k L^{(k)}(M(t))/k! \tag{8.6}$$

8.4.3 Generalized accelerated failure time (GAFT) frailty model

The accelerated failure time(AFT) model can be easily extended with frailty model due to the linear formation. Suppose the baseline survival function is defined as $S_0(t)$ with q-dimensional vector z_{ij}. It is usually a subset of x_{ij}. The model can be formulated with GAFT as

$$S_{X_{ij}}(t) = S_{0,z_{ij}}(e^{-x_{ij}^T\beta - v_i t}) \tag{8.7}$$

or equivalently,

$$y_{ij} = \log(t_{ij}) = x_{ij}^T\beta + v_i + \epsilon_{ij} \tag{8.8}$$

Now $x_{ij} = (1, x_{ij}^T)^T$ provides the intercept value. The corresponding vector is formulated as $\beta = (\beta_0, \beta^T)^T$. The heteroscedastic error can be estimated as ϵ_{ij}. It is independent of v_i, and $P(e^{\beta_0 + \epsilon_{ij}} > t|z_{ij}) = S_{0,z_{ij}}(t)$. It is defined as

$$\epsilon_{ij}|G_{z_{ij}} \sim G_{z_{ij}} \tag{8.9}$$

Now the term G_z is a probability measure defined on R for every $z \in X$. It is defined as a model for the entire collection of probability as $G_X = \{G_z : z \in X\}$. It allows us about smoothly change with the covariates z.

It can be formulated as

$$\beta \sim N_{p+1}(m_0, S_0)$$

$$G_z|\alpha, \sigma^2 \sim \text{LDTFP}_L(\alpha, \sigma^2), \alpha \sim \Gamma(a_0, b_0), \sigma^{-2} \sim \Gamma(a_\sigma, a_\sigma)$$

8.4.4 Illustration with leukemia data using R

A total of seven R packages are required to work Bayesian frailty model in R. Packages are "coda","survival","spBayesSurv","fields","BayesX","R2BayesX" and "spBayesSurv" respectively.   and

```
#Leukemia Data Using R

library("coda")
library("survival")
library("spBayesSurv")
library("fields")
library("BayesX")
library("R2BayesX")
library("spBayesSurv")
```

A total of n=1,043 patients leukemia data is considered. The dataset is available as LeukSurv data in "spBayesSurv" package. This illustration is about exploring the subject-specific variation after adjusting the factors like sex, white blood cell, Townsend score (TPI) and sex.

Now patients have belonged to a different district. It may be possible that subjective variation has occurred due to a native of the patients. In this context, the geostatistical and area wise models are fitted. Dataset is presented as

```
#Leukemia Data Illustration Using R

data("LeukSurv")
d <- LeukSurv[order(LeukSurv$district), ] head(d)
```

The outcome looks like

```
# R Output to Check Dataset

   time cens xcoord      ycoord     age sex wbc   tpi   district
   24   1    1    0.4123484 0.4233738 44  1   281.0 4.87  1
   62   3    1    0.3925028 0.4531422 72  1   0.0   7.10  1
   68   4    1    0.4167585 0.4520397 68  0   0.0   5.12  1
   128  9    1    0.4244763 0.4123484 61  1   0.0   2.90  1
   129  9    1    0.4145535 0.4520397 26  1   0.0   6.72  1
   163  15   1    0.4013230 0.4785006 67  1   27.9  1.50  1
```

Now another dataset "newngland" is called that is available in spBayesSurv.

```
#Newngland Data Illustration Using R

Newngland <- read.bnd(system.file("otherdata/newngland.bnd",
+package = "spBayesSurv"))
adj.mat <- bnd2gra(Newngland)
E <- diag(diag(adj.mat)) - as.matrix(adj.mat)
```

Thereafter district are sorted from the LeukSurv dataset. Finally, the adjacency matrix E is obtained as Next task is to assign a function to run the MCMC algorithm. A total of 5,000 burn-in scans are planned with nburn=5000. A final chain of 2,000 is fixed as nsave=2000. The thinning interval to run the MCMC is defined by nskip=4. A total of scans to be saved is defined as nsave. The predefined number of scans to be displayed on the screen is called by ndisplay.

```
#Simulation Size Specification

set.seed(1)
mcmc <- list(nburn = 5000, nsave = 2000, nskip = 4, ndisplay = 1000)
```

The prior information is assigned as prior. It is performed as transformed Bernstein polynomial (TBP) prior [38].

```
#Prior Information Specification

prior <- list(maxL = 4, a0 = 5, b0 = 1)
ptm <- proc.time()
```

Finally, the function is used to fit a generalized accelerated failure time frailty model. The function is frailtyGAFT available in spBayesSurv [39]. This function is useful for frailty modeling on cluster level time-to-event data. The outcome is assigned to res1. The variables like age, sex, wbc, and tpi are considered as covariates on time-to-event data modeling.

```
#Model Specification

res1    <-    frailtyGAFT(formula    =    Surv(time,    cens)    ~
age+sex+wbc+tpi+
baseline(age, sex, wbc, tpi) + frailtyprior("car" district),
data = d, mcmc = mcmc, prior = prior, Proximity = E)
(sfit1 <- summary(res1))
frailtyGAFT(formula = Surv(time, cens) ~ age + sex + wbc + tpi +
baseline(age, sex, wbc, tpi) + frailtyprior("car", district),
data = d, mcmc = mcmc, prior = prior, Proximity = E)
proc.time() - ptm
```

The posterior estimates for age, sex, WBC and tpi are obtained as 8.58, -0.05, -0.26, -0.00 and -0.06 respectively. The estimates obtained through Bayesian is presented with posterior estimates.

```
#R Output

Generalized accelerated failure time frailty model:
Call:
frailtyGAFT(formula = Surv(time, cens) ~ age + sex
 +wbc+tpi+baseline(age,sex,wbc,tpi)+frailtyprior("car",
    district), data = d, mcmc = mcmc, prior = prior,
Proximity = E)

Posterior means for regression coefficients:
          Mean    Median Std    95%HPD-Low  95%HPD-Upp
Intercept  8.58    8.60   0.28   7.98        9.14
age       -0.05   -0.05   0.00  -0.05       -0.04
sex       -0.26   -0.28   0.16  -0.53        0.06
wbc       -0.00   -0.00   0.00  -0.00       -0.00
tpi       -0.06   -0.06   0.01  -0.09       -0.02
Bayes factors for LDTFP covariate effects:
intercept age     sex    wbc    tpi  overall  normality
 130.95    11.62  1.26   14.01  0.48 7.88      994.86
```

The traceplot for age covariates can be generated through

```
#Model Diagnostics
traceplot(mcmc(res1beta[1,]))
```

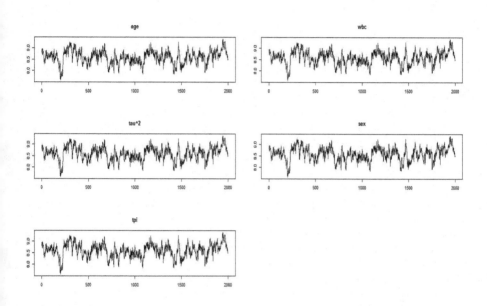

FIGURE 8.3: Trace plot of estimates.

Chapter 9

Relative Survival Analysis

Abstract

Relative survival is helpful to understand the more deaths due to cancer in comparison to the general population. It helps to determine the deaths due to cancer by eliminating other causes of mortality. However, it requires to define the causes of death. Even cancer patients may die due to other causes. The cancer registry data always influenced by other causes of mortality. It is required to define the causes of death rigorously. The application of relative survival is minimal only on cancer have low survival rates. Now the relative survival analysis by Bayesian counterpart is presented in the chapter. Cancer clinical trial data example is shown in this chapter. The definition of piecewise hazard function is presented. Further, the step to compute the piecewise hazard value is performed. This chapter will help to provide information that is difficult to address by conventional analysis. The computation of relative survival is presented by OpenBUG software, as a Bayesian counterpart. The methodology of relative survival by the multiplicative and additive model is presented.

9.1 Introduction

Survival analysis is the only tool to understand cancer disease severity. It is very much required to understand different progress in cancer care by applying the survival analysis. Now the cancer survival can be presented in different forms. Now the net cancer survival separates the impact of a cancer diagnosis on different survival, and it is useful statistics to explain the cancer prognosis. Net cancer survival defines the probability of surviving a cancer diagnosis in the absence of competing causes of death. Net survival is most often used by two technique, i.e., competing for risk and relative survival. Now, in this chapter, we will show the work with relative survival. The application of relative survival becomes useful in the National Cancer Institute's Surveillance, Epidemiology and End Results (SEER) the program. Relative survival estimates the percent of persons surviving by death adjusted for expected deaths by life table data. Now relative survival estimates the life expectancies for the US populations based on current age. In contrast, the expected survival of a population does not give us accurate information about the expected survival of a population of patients with a cancer diagnosis. Now the life tables cannot be generalized to all populations, and relative survival analysis is an alternative. However, it is required to have a reference population to perform relative survival. However, while the reference population is not available, the competing risk analysis is possible to apply. Relative survival used to compare the death of cancer patients in comparison to the general population. The documentation about the cause of death among cancer patients plays an important role. Thereafter, the comparison of the patients' death due to cancer is compared with the population. This helps to consider population-based studies where a large number of patients are followed through a longitudinal study. It is also important for clinical trials where more clinical information is present. This is a standard methodology in registry data analysis for cancer patients. The approach is about coupling the measured death information with general mortality data. It provides to obtain the disease-specific hazard. Perhaps, the practical application of relative survival analysis is relatively complex. Because the hazard rate also changes for different age and time. Commonly the population-based studies involved a large number of population with long-term follow-up. However, it is difficult to capture all types of clinical information for population-based long-term follow-up studies. It is difficult to capture all cause of death for a long-time follow-up study. The information about relapse, remission and progression are difficult to obtain in population-based studies. The cause of death is often unreliable or unavailable. Suppose a bone metastasis has occurred to a lung cancer patient. The cause of death is documented as bone cancer. The primary cancer is lung, and cause of death should be lung cancer. Sometimes cancer patients die due to chemotherapy-related severe toxicity. It is difficult to find the cause of death as specific cancer or drug toxicity. Even the actual information about the cause of death is present. It is often challenging to classify the cause of death due to cancer or not, the widely accepted approach to classifying the cause of death as due to cancer or not. The application of relative survival is not new [7]. It is used a long time in cancer registry data. The widely accepted approach is non-parametric survival curve comparison [40]. Recently, methodological extensions are carried in terms of the estimator [41, 42]. The net survival becomes an attractive choice as non-parametric estimator [43]. The detailed about the non-parametric procedure is well-documented [44].

9.2 Relative Survival Analysis

> #Definition of Relative Survival
>
> The relative survival is defined as
>
> $$S_R(t) = \frac{S_O(t)}{S_P(t)} \qquad (9.1)$$

This ratio helps to make a comparison of patients from the general population. Survival of the patients becomes very poor if the ratio is lesser than one. It is not obvious that the survival curve will be monotonously increasing [45]. The ratio can be used to compare the survival measures between two cohorts adjusted by different demographic variable. It is assumed that the overall hazard of each cancer patients can be defined as λ_{Oi}. It can be split into two parts as a hazard due to cancer(λ_{Ei}) and hazard present in the general population (λ_{Pi}). There is a gap between methodological development and practical application. Some methodological development is required on ad-hoc changes in the existing function. The relative survival analysis can be performed in R. The "resurv" is suitable enough to perform the different relative survival analysis. This function is useful toward importing the population tables through regression analysis. Futher, the individual level survival can be defined as

$$S_{E_i}(t) = \exp\{-\int_0^t \lambda_{E_i}(u)du\} = \frac{\exp\{-\int_0^t \lambda_{O_i}(u)du\}}{\exp\{-\int_0^t \lambda_{P_i}(u)du\}} \qquad (9.2)$$

Suppose a cohort size is N. The marginal relative survival ratio can be defined as

$$S_E(t) = \frac{1}{N}\sum_{i=1}^{N} S_{E_i}(t) \qquad (9.3)$$

Now the net survival is defined as

> #Definition of Net Survival
>
> $$S_R(t) = \frac{\frac{1}{N}\sum_{i=1}^{N} S_{O_i}(t)}{\frac{1}{N}\sum_{i=1}^{N} S_{P_i}(t)}; S_E(t) = \frac{\frac{1}{N}\sum_{i=1}^{N} S_{O_i}(t)}{\frac{1}{N}\sum_{i=1}^{N} S_{P_i}(t)} \qquad (9.4)$$

9.3   Data Methodology

Data of this illustrated work is obtained from Tata Memorial Hospital among patients treated between January 2012 and December 2015. Patients having Stage III and Stage IV treated with TKI were included in this study. The proven pathological disease like ECOG, PS indicator a 3-4 and previously untreated patients were considered in this study. A total of 630 patients (396 males, 234 females), with ages ranging from 2 to 87 (mean 60), diagnosed between 2011 and 2015 and followed until 2017 were considered in this work. The data consist of times in days from date of registration to death. Predictor variables include the Stage of the disease at diagnosis (1-4), the year of diagnosis (Yr), and the age at diagnosis (Age). The predictor variables are EGFR, Age, Stage, Diabetes and metastatic present or not. We are interested in comparing the survival between EGFR positive and negative.

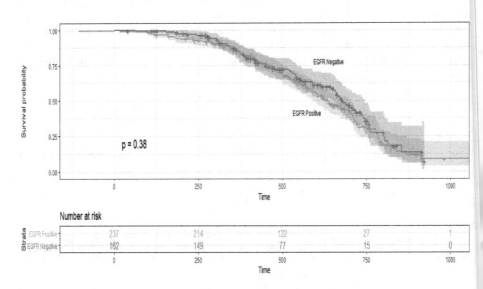

FIGURE 9.1: Survival comparison between EGFR postive and EGFR negative.

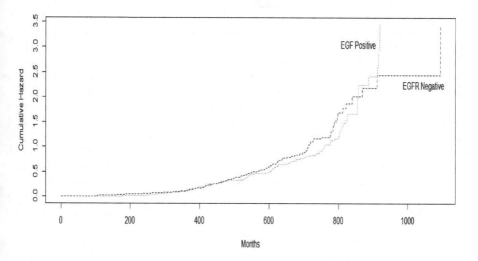

FIGURE 9.2: Cumulative survial curve between EGFR postive and EGFR negative.

9.4 Illustration with R

The individual expected survival of a cohort could be obtained through Relative Survival. The individual expected survival is required to make toward comparison on age and sex composition. The R package relsurv is useful to obtain relative survival based on population table. The population contains expected death rates from the calendar year, age, and sex.

```
#Relaive Survival by Survexp Function

library("survival")
haz  <-  survexp(OS~1,data=mydata,  rmap  =  list(year=year,
age=age1), method='individual.h')
```

This function is useful to obtain each individual's survival experience. For each individual, the total hazard experienced up to their observed death time or last follow-up time. This probability is used as a rescaled time value in the models.

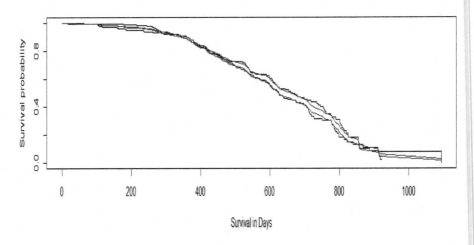

FIGURE 9.3: Survial comparison between EGFR postive and EGFR negative.

```
#Relaive Survival Using R
glm(mydata $ death ~ 1 + offset(log(haz)), family=poisson)
glm(mydata$ death ~mydata$EGFR+offset(log(haz)),family=poisson)
```

In the first model, a statistical test is performed. The intercept is considered as 0. It defined with the log-rank test of whether the observed group of the subject has equal survival to the baseline population or not. The second model is considered for an effect of variable x after adjusting with reference to sex and age. Different variables are combined in the rate table. It is useful to have a different dataset, to deal with the ramp. The rate table served to compute survexp.us and thereafter expected survival with reference to age and sex. The cohort group comparison is performed by the overall survival curve. The visual conclusion can be obtained through the survival curve. Survival curves can be compared through the "exact method".

```
#Relative Survival Analysis

library("survival")
haz <- survexp(OS~1, data=mydata,
rmap = list(year=year, age=age1),method="individual.h")
glm(mydata$death~1 + offset(log(haz)), family=poisson)
glm(mydata$death ~mydata$EGFR + offset(log(haz)),
family=poisson)
pfit<-coxph(Surv(OS,death>0) EGFR+Stage+Diabetes+
metapresent,data=mydata)
plot(survfit(Surv(OS,death>0)~EGFR, data=mydata),
ylab="Survival probability",xlab="Survival in Days",
main="Relative Surival of having EGFR positive",
mark.time=FALSE)
lines(survexp(~EGFR, ratetable=pfit, data=mydata),
col='purple')
```

```
# R output with Realtive Survival Analysis(Model 1)

Call:glm(formula = mydata$death~1+offset(log(haz)),
family = poisson)

Coefficients:
(Intercept)
    3.474

Degrees of Freedom: 629 Total (i.e. Null);  629 Residual
Null Deviance:      453.9
Residual Deviance: 453.9         AIC: 1086
```

```
# R Output with Realtive Survival Analysis(Model 2)

Call:glm(formula=mydata$death~mydata$EGFR+offset(log(haz)),
    family = poisson)

Coefficients:
(Intercept)  mydata$EGFR
    3.49530      -0.04192

Degrees of Freedom: 629 Total (i.e. Null);  628 Residual
Null Deviance:      453.9
Residual Deviance: 453.8         AIC: 1088
```

9.5   Piecewise Hazard Function

The survival quantification can be carried by the cumulative risk of survival. It is reliable toward treatment effect comparison [46, 47]. The goal is to quantify the survival benefit in a specific time interval. Suppose the entire time interval is $[0, \tau_k]$. Thereafter it canbe split into $\tau_1 - \tau_0, \tau_2 - \tau_1, ..., \tau_k - \tau_{k-1}$ and $0 = \tau_0 < \tau_1 < .... < \tau_k$. Similarly, the hazard is formulated as $0 = g_0 < g_1 < .... < g_k$ and $g_0 = 1$. Piecewise constant function is

$$h(t) = h_0 \sum_{l=0}^{k} \tau_l I_l(t) \text{ with } I_l(t) = 1 \text{ if } \tau_l \leq t \leq \tau_{l+1}, \text{otherwise } I_l(t) = 0 \quad (9.5)$$

Survival function can be defined as

$$S(t) = exp(-H(t)) \quad (9.6)$$

Cumuative hazard function is

$$H(t) = \int_0^t h(s)ds = h_0 \sum_{l=0}^{m} g_l \int_0^t I_l(s)ds \quad (9.7)$$

9.6   Piecewise Hazard testing

Since we have several hazard functions value at a different point, it is useful to compare different hazard, and it comes under multiple testing problem. Suppose the term $X_1, ...X_n$ gives independently identically distributed survival times, and it is defined with $C_1, ...C_n$ censoring time. It is assumed that as independently distributed of X. Pair of observation are $(T_i, \delta_i), i = 1, 2, ...n$, with minimal time point $T_i = min(X_i, C_i)$ and $i = 1$. If $\delta_i = 1$ if $X_i \leq C_i$ and zero otherwise. Now it is presented as $0 < \tau_0 < \tau_1 < ..... < \tau_k = \infty$. Let us assume that a total of change point is k, and the number of change points in the model is α_j. The value of the hazard function between the time point is τ_{j-1} and τ_j.

The log-likelihood function is presented as

$$\log L(\alpha_1, ..., \alpha_{k+1}, \tau_1, ...\tau_k) = \sum_{j=1}^{k+1} [X(\tau_j) - X(\tau_{j-1})] \log \alpha_j - \sum_{i=1}^{n} \sum_{j=1}^{k+1} \alpha_j (T_i \Lambda \tau_j - T_i \Lambda \tau_{j-1}) \quad (9.8)$$

Now $X(t) = \sum_{i=1}^{n} I(T \le t, \delta_i = 1)$ is presented as the number of death measured till time t. It is possible to make $\tau_j, j = 1, ...k$ as fixed and maximize it as $\tau_j, j = 1, ...k + 1$. The function can be formulated as

$$\tau_j = \frac{(X(\tau_j) - X(\tau_{j-1}))}{\sum_{i=1}^{n}(T_i \Lambda \tau_j - T_i \Lambda \tau_{j-1})I(T > \tau_{j-1})} \tag{9.9}$$

The likelihood for τ_j is expressed as

$$l(\tau_1, \tau_2, ..., \tau_k) = \sum_{j=1}^{k+1}\{X(\tau_j - X(\tau_{j-1})\}\log\frac{(X(\tau_j) - X(\tau_{j-1}))}{\sum_{i=1}^{n}(T_i \Lambda \tau_j - T_i \Lambda \tau_{j-1})I(T > \tau_{j-1})} \tag{9.10}$$

It is maximize with $l(\tau_1, \tau_2, ..., \tau_k)$ with respect to $\tau_j.j = 1, ..., k$ and insert the obtained values back to $\hat{\tau}_j, j = 1, ..., k + 1$ for MLEs of α_j. Now it is required to test the changes of τ_j. The hypothesis can be performed as $H_0 : \tau_{j_1} - \tau_{j_2} = 0$. Now different factors can be considered to prepare τ_j. Now τ_{j_1} and τ_{j_2} are independent in nature.

It is explored that τ_{j_1} and τ_{j_2} are independent in nature [48]. The Wald-test is performed with

$$X_w = \frac{(\hat{\tau}_{k-1} - \hat{\tau}_k)^2}{var(\hat{\tau}_{k-1} - \hat{\tau}_k)} \tag{9.11}$$

It can be formulated with chi-quare test statistics with one degree of freedom under null hypothesis. The R function is defined as WaldTest(), to perform the test statistics.

```
#R Code to Run Relative Survival

WaldTest= function (L)
{
WaldTest = numeric (3)
names (WaldTest) = c("W","df","value")
r = dim (L)[1]
W = ((tau1-tau2)^2)/v
W = as.numeric(W)
pval=1-pchisq(W,1)
WaldTest[1] = W; WaldTest[2] = r; WaldTest[3]=pval
WaldTest
}#End function WaldTest
LL = rbind(c(1, -1)); LLthetahat = c(1, 1)
```

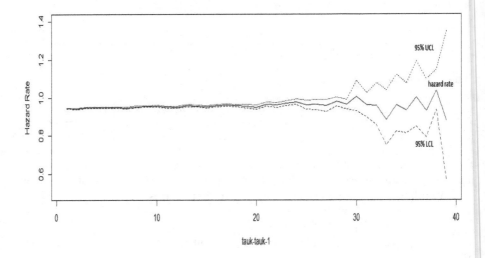

FIGURE 9.4: Piecewise hazard rate estimates comparison for different survival duration.

9.7   Piecewise Hazard Function Analysis

The prostate cancer data obtained from the Surveillance, Epidemiology, and End Results (SEER) Program (www.seer.cancer.gov) Public-Use Data (1973–2015), with a follow-up until December 2015. Dataset provides the incidence and survival information of those patients. Causes of death among patients are included in this dataset. cause of death due to other reasons are excluded from the dataset. Now patients died to prostrate cancer and censored are included.

9.8   Different Relative Survival Analysis Package with R

9.8.1   flexrsurv

This package is useful to allow to model non-linear and non-proportional effects using splines. It includes both non proportional and non linear effects.

#R Package Flexsurv for Relative Survival

```
library("flexrsurv")
library("relsurv")
data(rdata)
data(slopop)
rdata$iage<-findInterval(rdata$age ×365.24+rdata$time,
attr(slopop,"cutpoints")[[1]])
data$iyear<-findInterval(rdata$year+rdata$time,
attr(slopop, "cutpoints")[[2]])
therate <- rep(-1, dim(rdata)[1])
for( i in 1:dim(rdata)[1]){
therate[i] <- slopop[rdata$iage[i], rdata$iyear[i],
rdata$sex[i]] } rdata$slorate <- therate
rdata$sex01 <- rdata$sex -1
fit <- flexrsurv(Surv(time,cens) ~ sex01+
NLL(age, Knots=60, Degree=3,
Boundary.knots = c(24, 95)),
rate=slorate, data=rdata,
knots.Bh=1850, # one interior knot at 5 years
degree.Bh=3,
Max_T=5400,
Spline ="b-spline",
initbyglm=TRUE,
initbands=seq(0, 5400, 100),
int_meth="BANDS",
bands=seq(0, 5400, 50) )
summary(fit)
```

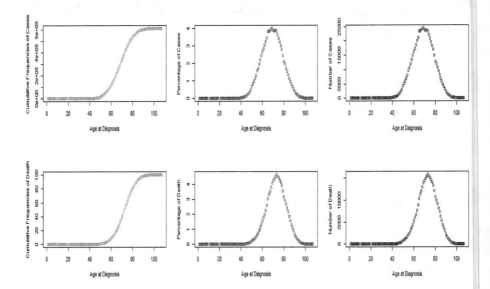

FIGURE 9.5: Different age wise cancer diagnosis, prostate cancer case distribution.

```
#Outcome of Flexrsurv Function

Coefficients:
Estimate Std. Error z value Pr(>|z|)
Baseline hazard:1 -9.3669 1.9478 -4.809 1.52e-06 ***
Baseline hazard:2 -10.8062 1.9569 -5.522 3.35e-08 ***
Baseline hazard:3 -10.6876 2.1408 -4.992 5.96e-07 ***
Baseline hazard:4 -10.7724 2.2308 -4.829 1.37e-06 ***
Baseline hazard:5 -10.5813 2.6117 -4.051 5.09e-05 ***
sex01 0.6852 0.1858 3.687 0.000227 ***
NLL(age):1 -0.6171 2.7501 -0.224 0.822446
NLL(age):2 1.6521 1.6531 0.999 0.317608
NLL(age):3 0.9809 2.5093 0.391 0.695865
NLL(age):4 2.3640 2.4392 0.969 0.332446
---

Signif. codes: 0 '***' 0.001 '**' 0.01 '*' 0.05 '.' 0.1 ' ' 1
Log-likelihood: -4781.327
```

9.8.2 relsurv

The relsurv package is useful to analyzing the relative survival data. It includes relative survival ratio, crude mortality, multiplicative regression model.

```
#R Package "Relsurv" for Relative Survival

library("relsurv")
data(slopop)
data(rdata)
rs.surv(Surv(time,cens)~sex,rmap=list(age=age×365.241),
ratetable=slopop,data=rdata)
d <- rs.surv.rsadd(fit,newdata=data.frame(sex=1,
age=65,year=as.date("1Jul1982"))
fit <- rsadd(Surv(time,cens) sex+age+year,
rmap=list(age=age×365.241),
ratetable=slopop,data=rdata,int=c(0:10,15))
plot(d,xscale=365.241)
```

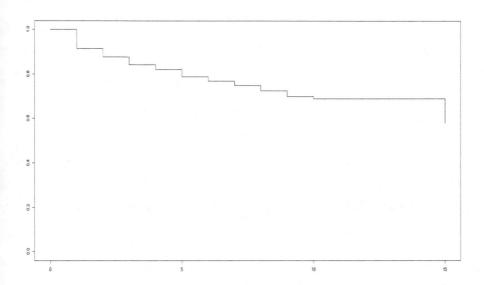

FIGURE 9.6: R package "relsurv" on r Relative Survival.

9.8.3   survexp.fr

This package is useful to obtain the Relative survival. Function "survexp_plot" avalible in "survexp.fr" is helpful to obtain the relative survival plot. The illustration given below.

```
#R Package "Survexp.fr" is Useful for Relative Survival

library("survexp.fr")
attach(data.example)
survexp_plot(futime, status, age, sex, entry_date)
```

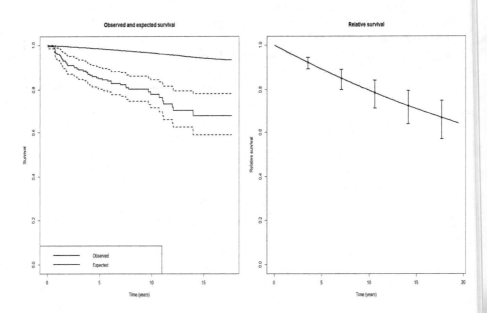

FIGURE 9.7: Survival plot obtained by survexp function.

TABLE 9.1: Piecewise hazard ratio estimates in different survival intervals in months

Interval	τ_1	τ_2	Hazard Ratio	95%Confidence Interval	Wald -Statistics	P -value
1	0	12	0.94	(0.94,0.94)	0.000	0.989
2	13	24	0.94	(0.94,0.94)	0.180	0.671
3	25	36	0.95	(0.94,0.95)	0.002	0.964
4	37	48	0.94	(0.94,0.95)	0.001	0.979
5	49	60	0.95	(0.94,0.95)	0.000	1
6	61	72	0.95	(0.94,0.95)	0.003	0.96
7	73	84	0.94	(0.94,0.95)	0.120	0.729
8	85	96	0.95	(0.95,0.95)	0.001	0.974
9	97	108	0.95	(0.95,0.96)	0.000	0.985
10	109	120	0.95	(0.95,0.96)	0.018	0.893
11	121	132	0.95	(0.94,0.95)	0.000	0.988
12	133	144	0.95	(0.94,0.95)	0.021	0.883
13	145	156	0.95	(0.95,0.96)	0.001	0.975
14	157	168	0.95	(0.95,0.96)	0.010	0.918
15	169	180	0.95	(0.94,0.95)	0.005	0.943
16	181	192	0.95	(0.95,0.96)	0.003	0.958
17	193	204	0.96	(0.95,0.97)	0.002	0.965
18	205	216	0.95	(0.95,0.96)	0.001	0.977
19	217	228	0.95	(0.94,0.96)	0.005	0.943
20	229	240	0.95	(0.94,0.96)	0.043	0.836
21	241	252	0.96	(0.95,0.97)	0.001	0.973
22	253	264	0.96	(0.95,0.97)	0.007	0.932
23	265	276	0.97	(0.95,0.98)	0.002	0.964
24	277	288	0.97	(0.96,0.99)	0.004	0.949
25	289	300	0.96	(0.94,0.98)	0.000	0.997
26	301	312	0.96	(0.93,0.99)	0.000	0.987
27	313	324	0.96	(0.92,0.99)	0.023	0.878
28	325	336	0.98	(0.95,1.00)	0.002	0.967
29	337	348	0.96	(0.94,0.99)	0.010	0.922
30	349	360	1.00	(0.93,1.09)	0.051	0.821
31	361	372	0.96	(0.90,1.02)	0.000	0.099
32	373	384	0.95	(0.85,1.07)	0.041	0.839
33	385	396	0.88	(0.75,1.04)	0.031	0.861
34	397	408	0.96	(0.82,1.12)	2.430	0.119
35	409	420	0.93	(0.81,1.07)	0.005	0.938
36	421	432	1.00	(0.84,1.19)	Inf	0
37	433	444	0.93	(0.79,1.09)	0.008	0.926
38	445	456	1.03	(0.93,1.15)	0.007	0.93
39	457	468	0.87	(0.57,1.34)	inf	0

TABLE 9.2: Piecewise hazard ratio estimates in different survival intervals in months for grade I

Interval	τ_1	τ_2	Hazard Ratio	95%Confidence Interval	Wald -Statistics	P -value
1	0	12	0.94	(0.93,0.94)	0.01	0.93
2	13	24	0.91	(0.88,0.95)	0	0.98
3	25	36	0.91	(0.88,0.95)	0.71	0.4
4	37	48	0.92	(0.89,0.95)	0.15	0.7
5	49	60	0.88	(0.84,0.92)	0.09	0.77
6	61	72	0.89	(0.82,0.97)	0.09	0.76
7	73	84	0.9	(0.81,0.99)	0	0.99
8	85	96	0.9	(0.83,0.97)	0.01	0.92
9	97	108	0.9	(0.83,0.98)	0.12	0.73
10	109	120	0.88	(0.83,0.93)	0.44	0.51
11	121	132	0.93	(0.88,0.98)	0.04	0.84
12	133	144	0.91	(0.86,0.95)	0.01	0.91
13	145	156	0.92	(0.88,0.95)	0.02	0.89
14	157	168	0.9	(0.87,0.94)	0.04	0.89
15	169	180	0.91	(0.88,0.94)	0.02	0.85
16	181	192	0.93	(0.91,0.96)	0.61	0.88
17	193	204	0.95	(0.92,0.98)	0	0.44
18	205	216	0.95	(0.92,0.98)	0	0
20	229	240	0.93	(0.90,0.95)	0.1	0.33
21	241	252	0.97	(0.95,1.00)	0.02	0.75
22	253	264	0.94	(0.92,0.97)	0.08	0.88
23	265	276	0.98	(0.95,1.01)	0	0.77
24	277	288	0.96	(0.93,1.00)	0.02	0.96
25	289	300	0.98	(0.94,1.02)	0	0.89
26	301	312	0.96	(0.92,1.00)	0.01	0.95
27	313	324	0.98	(0.93,1.04)	0.05	0.94
28	325	336	0.95	(0.89,1.01)	0	0.82
29	337	348	0.95	(0.86,1.05)	0.02	0.1
30	349	360	0.99	(0.91,1.08)	0	0.99
31	361	372	1	(0.90,1.11)	0.03	0.85
32	373	384	0.94	(0.81,1.09)	0.03	0.85
33	385	396	0.84	(0.66,1.06)	0.03	0.86
34	397	408	0.97	(0.77,1.22)	0.03	0.86
35	409	420	0.87	(0.71,1.07)	0.02	0.88
36	421	432	1.11	(0.60,2.05)	Inf	0
37	433	444	0.21	(0.00,0.38)	0.1	0.75
38	445	456	0.88	(0.41,1.90)	0.17	0.68

9.9 Discussion

Relative survival analysis can help us to provide information that is difficult to address by conventional analysis. It is really useful to adopt a conventional analysis of a better therapeutic effect comparison. We illustrate the application through OpenBUG software. It is performed as a Bayesian counterpart. The methodology of relative survival by the multiplicative and additive model is well-elaborated [49]. The application of relative survival at an individual level is also documented [50]. The application of relative survival is very limited only on cancer have low survival rates. A good explanation about relative and net survival is well-documented [45]. Cause-specific survival can be used toward median duration survival estimates. However, it is applicable in relative survival. The hazard function estimates are developed through predictive scoring. The treatment effect can be compared through different age interval by piecewise hazard. It is also applicable in health policy implementation. This chapter provides the importance of relative survival, and piecewise estimates of hazard function are feasible to use to develop prediction score as well. It will provide us with another dimension about the establishment of therapeutic effect. It may be important toward health policy decision. This work will help to understand the hazard function at a different time point interval.

Part III

Bayesian in Longitudinal Data Analysis

Chapter 10

Longitudinal Data Analysis

Abstract

To describe different types of statistical tool and analytical approach for longitudinal data analysis in oncology. A different aspect of longitudinal study design is presented. The Bayesian counterpart to perform longitudinal data analysis in oncology is furnished. The Bayesian estimation of a balanced longitudinal model with ARMA(1) the structure is provided. Another covariance structure like compound symmetry is explained with R packages. Finally, A study is presented to compare the Quality of Life in palliative patients treated with two chemotherapeutic arms. It provides the best arm to maintain better QoL among treated patients. The observations are taken repeatedly for each patient during treatment. The application of the mixed effect model is implemented.

10.1 Introduction

In oncology, conventionally the endpoints are considered as a clinical outcome as clinical efficacy. Conventionally, clinical efficacy is defined by overall survival (OS). Similarly, biological efficacy also considered through disease-free survival (DFS). The OS is the gold standard in any oncology trial. Perhaps, it is difficult to consider for any clinical benefits. The therapeutic effect becomes more attractive if it can provide a better quality of life (QoL). The QoL always measured in a repeated manner through patients experience. The QoL measured as a standard questionnaire. After that, the comparison of QoL between the treatment arm provides the best effective treatment. The QoL measures repeated outcomes over time. In a conventional randomized controlled trial, the baseline QoL assessed and followed up longitudinally. In repeated QoL, the same individual subjects observed, and observations are correlated. The traditional statistical approach for analyzing such data is not suitable enough. In this context, this chapter dedicated to mixed effect modeling to Analysis of QoL data. The Linear mixed effect is a method to deal with repeatedly measured QoL. Currently, the health-related quality of life (HRQoL) becomes an important parameter. Longitudinal QoL data are widely adopted to explore cancer progression. It shows that whether the change measured over time is related to socio-economic factors, age at onset, education and other genetic factors. However, the change of QoL over time across individuals is logical. This data analysis is not straightforward. The well-appreciated method for longitudinal data analysis is random or mixed effect modeling. There are several biostatistical application of longitudinal data. Both in epidemiological and clinical filed. The term longitudinal defined as repeatedly measured observations of the same individual. The focus of this work is to determine whether changes over time occurred or not. The focus of this work is about Bayesian methods for longitudinal data analysis through the mixed effect model.

10.2   Advantages of Longitudinal Analysis

(I) Prospective ascertainment of exposure.
(II) Separation of time effects.
(III) Incident events are recorded.
(IV) Measurement of individual change in outcomes.

10.3   Limitation of Longitudinal Analysis

(I) Participant follow-up.
(II) Correlated data.
(III) Time-varying covariates.

10.4   Mixed Effect Model

The relation between outcome and associated factors are explored by statistical modeling. The widely adopted statistical model is the linear model. Further, this linear model can be separated into fixed and random effect. The parameters linked with an entire population is considered as a fixed effect. However, the parameters changes individually are considered a random effect. A model consisted of the fixed and random parameter is defined as the mixed-effect model. Suppose that patients QOL is measured repeatedly. The repeated measurements are defined as y_{ij}. The ith individuals jth time point measurement is defined as y_{ij}. Now if the maximum number of visits are defined as m then $j = 1, ..., m_i$. Similarly, a total of n sample data is defined as $i = 1, ..., n$. The mean parameter linked with each measurement is μ_{ij}. Now the term μ_{ij} changes from different situations. For example, the presence of two time period ($j = 1, 2$) says the estimation of μ_{i1}, μ_{i2} will vary. The simple relation can be obtained as $\mu_{ij} = \alpha \mu_{i,j-1}$.

The model can be settled as

$$y_{ij}|\mu_{ij} \sim \mathrm{N}(\mu_{ij}, \sigma^2) \tag{10.1}$$

$$\mu_{ij} = x_{ij}^T \beta + z_{ij}^T b_i \tag{10.2}$$

The term $x_{ij}^T \beta$ is a linear predictor. The random effect component is $z_{ij}^T b_i$ for the ith individuals jth time point measurement. The covariance matrix is presented as V_i.

In a Bayesian framework, the prior distributions required to assigned. The prior dustrubution for β and b_i is assumed. It is feasible to assign b_i as $N(0, \tau^2)$. Further the prior value τ^2 can be assigned as IG$(1, 0.0260)$. The likelihood can be written as

$$\prod_{i,j} p(Y_{ij}|t_{ij}, b_i) \tag{10.3}$$

Now it can be assumed that $p(Y_{ij}|t_{ij}, b_i) = \mathrm{N}(\mu_{ij}, \sigma^2)$ and

$$\mu_{ij} = \beta_0 + \beta_1.t_{ij} + b_{0,i} \tag{10.4}$$

It is required to assign the prior distributions for b_i, β_0, β_1, and σ^2. The posterior distribution is presented as

$$\prod_{i,j} p(Y_{ij}|t_{ij}, b_i, \sigma^2, \tau^2) \prod_i \pi(b_i, \tau^2)\pi(\beta_0)\pi(\beta_1)\pi(\sigma^2)\pi(\tau^2) \tag{10.5}$$

10.5 Different R Packages for Longitudinal Data Analysis

Longitudinal data always measured to understand disease progression and process. However, it depends on the number of longitudinal observations tumour progression measured by growth or recurrence. The "growcurves" package available in R is suitable to perform the hierarchical Bayesian modeling for dependence among subjects, by continued and combined therapy. It works by Dirichlet process before random-effect modeling. It brings the information to estimate as flexible and non-parametric. A different statistical package like

MLwiN is useful for parametric hierarchical modeling. DP prior one random effect model is applicable by "DPpackage" . Challenges to work with missing value, explore different quality criterion and the graphical interface is nicely handled by "kml" package. The likelihood clustering distance metric performed by "kmlcov" package works through the generalized linear model the recursive separation of linear and nonlinear mixed effect performed by "longRPart2" package.

10.6   Random-Effect Model with R

A dedicated team for R (R Core Team 2019) provides the R package lme4 to work with linear mixed effect model [51]. The function is known as lme4. The generalized linear mixed models and nonlinear mixed models are possible to work with lme4 function. The term mixed is used to accommodate the fixed and random effect. In this chapter, we discussed Bayesian application with linear mixed effect model.

The alterative of lme4 is nlme that is available in R for mixed-effect modeling (Pinheiro, Bates, DebRoy, Sarkar, and R Core Team 2015). However, lme4 is efficient toward the complex situation. It is simple to perform on random effect models. It is easy to perform by likelihood function on random effect. The package "nlme" is compatible to work with residuals and the residuals generated due to heteroscedasticity and autocorrelation structure.

The packages used to work with specific functions in R. These functions developed with logic, statistics, probability, and mathematical programming. Few essential and basic functions automatically installed in R. The specific function can only work through the installation of the package. There are several thousand packages available in R to work with the specialized problem. The list of packages is available in http://cran.r-project.org. These packages can also be downloaded from: http://cran.r-project.org. In R console this packages can also be installed by using the packages pulldown menu in R. The lme4 package is useful to work with mixed effect model. A drop-down menu can install this package. After that, this package is required to load by running the library(lme4) in R console.

10.6.1   bayeslongitudinal

This function is used to obtain the longitudinal regression model by Bayesian methodology. There are two functions, i.e., mhsc and mharmal1. The mharmal1 is used for autoregressive modeling and mhsc for compound symmetry structure. Both the function is illustrated below:

Bayesian Estimation of a Balanced Longitudinal Model with ARMA(1) Structure

```
library("bayeslongitudinal")
attach(Dental)
Y=as.vector(distance)
X=as.matrix(cbind(1,age))
mharma11(Y,X,27,4,c(1,1),0.5,0.5,1,1,1,1,500,50)
```

mharma11(Data, Matriz, individuos, tiempos, betai, rhoi, gammai, beta1i, beta2i, beta1j, beta2j, iteraciones, burn).

Data A=vector with the observations of the response variable.

Matriz=The model design matrix.

individuos=A numerical value indicating the number of individuals in the study.

tiempos=A numerical value indicating the number of times observations were repeated.

betai=A vector with the initial values of the vector of regressors.

rhoi= A numerical value with the initial value of the correlation for rho.

gammai= A numerical value with the initial value of the correlation for phi.

beta1i= A numerical value with the shape parameter of a beta apriori distribution of rho.

beta2i= A numerical value with the scaling parameter of a beta apriori distribution of rho.

beta1j= A numerical value with the shape parameter of a beta apriori distribution of phi.

beta2j= A numerical value with the scaling parameter of a beta apriori distribution of phi.

iteraciones= A numerical value with the number of iterations that will be applied the algorithm MCMC.

burn= Number of iterations that are discarded from the chain.

```
# Bayesian Estimation of a Balanced Longitudinal Model with Com-
pound Symmetry Structure

library("bayeslongitudinal")
attach(Dental)
Y=as.vector(distance)
X=as.matrix(cbind(1,age))
mhsc(Y,X,27,4,c(1,1),0.5,1,1,500,50)
mhsc(Data, Matriz, individuos, tiempos, betai, rhoi, beta1i, beta2i,
iteraciones, burn)
```
Data A=vector with the observations of the response variable.
Matriz=The model design matrix.
individuos=A numerical value indicating the number of individuals in the study.
tiempos=A numerical value indicating the number of times observations were repeated.
betai=A vector with the initial values of the vector of regressors.
rhoi=A numerical value with the initial value of the correlation.
beta1i=A numerical value with the shape parameter of a beta apriori distribution of rho.
beta2i=A numerical value with the scaling parameter of a beta apriori distribution of
rho=iteraciones numerical value with the number of iterations that will be applied the algorithm.
MCMC=burn Number of iterations that are discarded from the chain.

10.7   Illustration with Quality of Life Using OpenBUGS

A study was performed in India to compare the Quality of Life in palliative patients treated with two chemotherapeutic arms. The study about compares the best arm to maintain better QoL among treated patients. The observations are taken repeatedly for each patient during treatment. This study has required the application of the mixed effect model. The data illustrated in Table 10.1. the overall data trend plotted through the spaghetti plot. Spaghetti plot is a widely used tool in longitudinal data plotting. The R package "ggplot" can be used to plot in R.

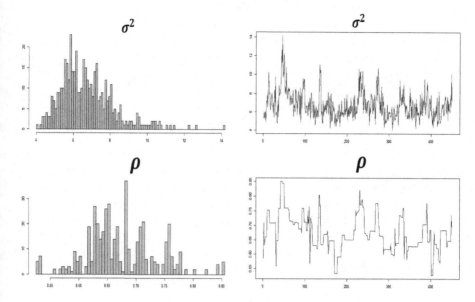

FIGURE 10.1: Bayesian estimation with compound symmetry structure.

```
library("ggplot2")
mydata<-data.frame(ID,painscore,visit,Arm)
p <- ggplot(data = mydata, aes(x = time,y=painscore,group=ID))
p + geomline()
```

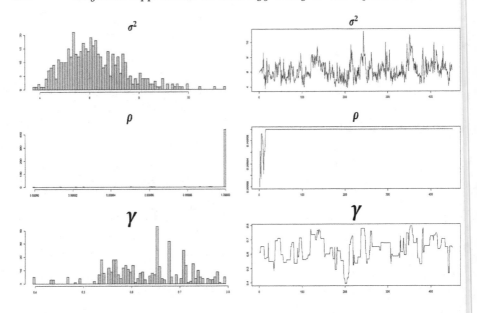

FIGURE 10.2: Bayesian estimation with ARMA(1) structure.

```
# Pain Score Illustrated Data

ID painscore Visit    Arm      ID painscore Visit    Arm
1   13.18    1    A             4   20.75    1    A
1   17.32    2    A             4   30.74    2    A
1   29.55    3    A             4   23.24    3    A
1   34.53    4    A             4   34.17    4    A
1   23.78    5    A             4   24.93    5    A
1   20.18    6    A             4   32.94    6    A
1   30.63    7    A             4   23.51    7    A
2   27.46    1    B             5   16.90    1    B
2   15.63    2    B             5   24.23    2    B
2   26.45    3    B             5   20.03    2    B
2   14.62    4    B             5   27.03    4    B
2   29.15    5    B             5   20.09    5    B
2   29.53    6    B             5   29.49    6    B
2   35.14    7    B             5   24.23    7    B
3   39.10    1    B             6   18.62    1    B
3   20.98    2    B             6   25.08    2    B
3   09.62    3    B             6   16.80    2    B
3   29.98    4    B             6   17.73    4    B
3   23.60    5    B             6   20.02    5    B
3   30.95    6    B             6   11.96    6    B
3   27.28    7    B             6   39.44    7    B
```

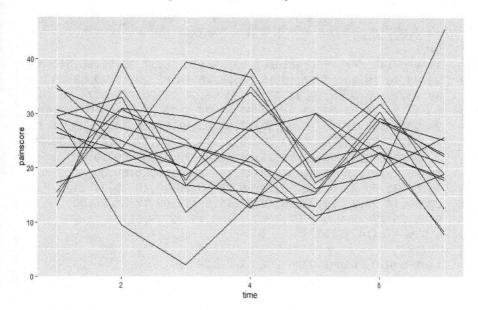

FIGURE 10.3: Longitudinal profile plot obtained by Spaghetti plot.

```
# Bayesian Mixed Effect Model in OpenBUGS

model {
for (i in 1:n) {
for (j in 1:K) {
mu[i,j] <- m + a[i]
y[i,j]~ dnorm( mu[i,j], tau )
}
a[i] ~ dnorm( 0, tau.a)
}
m~ dnorm(0.0,0.001)  #Define prior distribution of m
tau~dgamma(0.001,0.001)#Define prior distribution of tau
tau.a~dgamma(0.001,0.001)#Define prior distribution of tau.a
s2<- 1/tau # Define prior value for s2
s2.a<- 1/tau.a  # Define prior value for s2.a
ts2<- s2+s2.a  # Define value for ts2
cor<- s2.a/ts2  # calculate correaltion coefficient
s<-sqrt(s2)
s.a<- sqrt(s2.a)
for(i in 1:n) {
for(j in 1:K){
res[i,j]<- y[i,j]-mu[i,j]
}}
R2<-1-pow(sd(res[1:n,1:K])/sd(y[1:n,1:K]),2)
}
```

```
# Pain Score Illustrated Data

DATA
list(n=14, K=7,y=structure(.Data=c(13.18,17.32,29.55,34.53,
23.78,20.18,30.63,27.46,15.63,26.45,14.62,29.15,29.53,35.14,
39.10,20.98,9.62,29.44,23.60,30.95,27.28,20.75,30.74,23.24,
34.17,24.93,32.94,23.51,16.90,24.23,2.03,27.03,20.09,29.49,
24.23,18.62,25.08,16.80,17.73,20.02,11.96,39.44,15.59,21.12,
13.63,33.99,12.74,26.82,20.28,27.95,13.01,27.19,34.90,38.22,
22.25,36.68,12.98,15.71,23.14,21.09,30.17,30.09,10.30,
36.75,15.31,16.35,21.38,18.44,11.39,17.33,28.60,30.38,
33.50,31.80,22.62,19.50,22.95,28.68,29.28,18.75,24.31,
22.89,14.33,25.12,22.60,12.62,15.89,19.03,18.36,25.80,
8.39,25.17,22.21,45.62,7.82,17.88,19.02,20.87)
,.Dim = c(14, 7)))
INITS
list(m=0.0, tau=1.0)
```

10.8   Result

The application of longitudinal data in oncology research arises several times [52, 53, 54, 55, 56, 57, 54]. In epidemiological and clinical setup, both the case it is possible to occur. The mixed-effect model is used to show whether the changes in measurement over time individual level or group level as well. If the group level measurement difference occurs, then it is significant or not. The simple application of a mixed effect model is about a group of patients comparison between two time periods. The Bayesian method in longitudinal data presented in this chapter. The posterior mean of changes in pain score obtained with 23.11. The results also present individual variation and group-wise variation. The Analysis executed with 20,000 observations for the simulation, with the burn-in of 1,000 and a refresh of 100. The posterior distributions of within- and between-subject variabilities are observed through (σ_a^2 and σ^2, respectively) respectively. The trace plots for all these parameters given below. The OpenBUGS gives the trace plots. It shows the variation result for each parameter during the simulation.

TABLE 10.1: Posterior estimates obtained are presented

Parameter	Posterior mean	SD	2.5%	97.5%
μ	23.11	1.24	21.33	24.92
cor	0.02	0.05	0.00	0.15
τ	0.015	0.00	0.01	0.02
τ_a	95.15	275.6	0.09	917.30
σ_a	0.86	1.36	0.03	3.312
σ_a^2	2.61	26.15	0.00	10.97
$\sigma^2 + \sigma_a^2$	3.47	27.51	0.03	14.282
σ	8.08	0.60	7.00	9.34

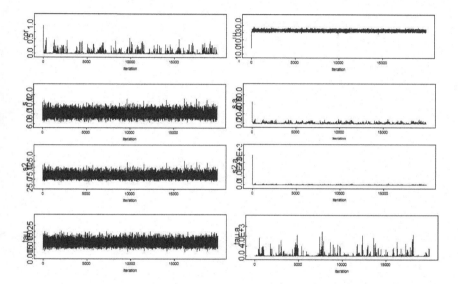

FIGURE 10.4: Trace plot of regression estimates obtained by 20,000 iterations.

Chapter 11

Missing Data Analysis

Abstract

The occurrence of missing data is common in any experimental field of research. Oncology research is not exceptional. Patients follow-up visits often occur. The follow-up visits raise the chance of appearance of missing observations. Missing observation seriously affects statistical inference. This chapter is about presenting a Bayesian technique to handle the missing data analysis. The objective is to obtain the best statistical inference in the presence of missing data.

11.1   Introduction

There is a different definition of missing data. Suppose the ith individuals jth time point measurement is defined as Y_{ij}. Now i could take a value from 1 to N. N is the sample size. Similarly, j can take any value from 0 to a maximum number of visits. Now another term R_{ij} as an indicator to represent the missing observation. If Y_{ij} is missing then $R_{ij} = 0$. If Y_{ij} is present then $R_{ij} = 1$. The term R_{ij} can be defined as the probability

$$P(R|Y_{\text{obs}}, Y_{\text{miss}}, \eta) \qquad (11.1)$$

η is the unknow parameter linked with missing.
Y_{obs} are the portion of the $n \times n$ matrix of Y that are present.
Y_{miss} are the portion of the $n \times n$ matrix of Y that are missing.

11.2   Different Types of Missing Data

11.2.1   Missing completely at random (MCAR)

The simplest form to define the type of missing data is called as missing completely at random (MCAR).

$$P(R|Y_{\text{obs}}, Y_{\text{miss}}, \eta) = P(R|\eta) \tag{11.2}$$

While the probability of missing data is independent of the observed data. If the missing data is unrelated to the observed data, for example, the patients missed his follow-up visit due to a hurricane of that day. The type of missing will be defined as MCAR.

However, if the same person missed the visit due to severe pain in his body. The patient is a subject of treatment outcome. Pain may occur due to dose toxicity. The missing data due to pain appearance will not be considered as MCAR. This MCAR do not affect the biasedness of the analysis. The power of the analysis indeed reduced, but it does not incline the bias in the dataset.

11.2.2   Missing at random (MAR)

The alternative form of MCAR is defined as missing at random (MAR).

$$P(R|Y_{\text{obs}}, Y_{\text{miss}}, \eta) = P(R|Y_{\text{obs}}, R|\eta) \tag{11.3}$$

The probability of the missing information is dependent only on the observed data. Data imputation technique is required to perform to overcome the missing information. Simple regression technique is useful to overcome the missing observation. It can be considered as ignorable missing.

11.2.3   Missing not at random (NMAR)

The third alternative is defined as missing not at random (NMAR). For example, a person having severe chemo response toxicity is less likely to fulfil the quality of life (QOL) questionnaires than others. This type of missing data is known as NMAR. The mean response of QOL obtained from missing data will be biased enough.

$$P(R|Y_{\text{obs}}\theta, \eta) = P(R|Y_{\text{obs}}, \eta)P(Y_{\text{obs}}|\theta) \tag{11.4}$$

If θ represents the vector of parameters for the distribution of Y. It shows that the inference for θ is based on the likelihood function, and it depends on the observed data. The likelihood is defined as

$$L(\theta|Y_{\text{obs}}) \propto P(Y_{\text{obs}}|\theta) \tag{11.5}$$

The Bayesian approach helps in this context. The likelihood is multiplied with the prior value of θ. The application of Bayes helped to obtain the posterior value of θ. Bayes's theorem is the posterior density of *theta*. Now the posterior estimate of θ can be obtained as

$$\pi(\theta|Y) = cL(Y|\theta)\pi(\theta) \tag{11.6}$$

The term c is used as normalizing constant and the likelihood function is presented as

$$L(Y|\theta) = f(Y|\theta) \tag{11.7}$$

The density is measured by f. The predicted density of the future observations is Z

$$g(z|y) \propto \int_{\Omega} f(z|\theta)\pi(\theta|y)d\theta \tag{11.8}$$

The integration is taken with respect to the parameter space Ω. The Bayesian method for missing data is helping to identify distributions for all the parameters. The parameters are assumed as the prior distribution. Both response and covariate can be imputed through the Bayesian method. The imputation is performed through prior distribution. Bayesian methods are free to impute data without any statistical inference. There are different method exists like Full Bayesian, maximum likelihood through Bayesian technique.

11.3 Different Softwares

There are different software to handle missing data in oncology research. The PROC MI is available is SAS to work with multiple imputation techniques for missing data. Perhaps, the normally distributed data is suitable to work with SAS. The right-censored data is not suitable to imputed through PROC MI. The OpenBUGS is an application software for the Bayesian analysis of complex statistical models. It works through Markov chain Monte Carlo (MCMC) methods. The missing data imputation technique can be easily performed in OpenBUGS. This software also works well with R. The R2OpenBUGS or BRugs packages are available in R to jointly work for further analysis.

11.4 Illustration with Lung Cancer Data

We consider data of Head and neck cancer conducted by the Tata Memorial Centre. The results of this study were reported by Noronha [58]. The palliative chemotherapy patients were selected in this study. Cetuximab is a costly chemotherapeutic drug. Only a total of 30 patients could afford this drug. The quality of life (QOL) data is presented among those patients. Similarly, another group of the cohort (n=40) is treated with cisplatin therapy. Data is filled with European Organisation for Research and Treatment of Cancer(EORTC) QOL questionnaire. The primary objective of this study was to compare the QOL between Cisplatin and Cetuximab arm. Presence of missing data is handled by Bayesian methodology. The imputation technique is performed to obtain the missing data. The comparison between treatment effect on repeated measurements is presented in Chapter 9. This chapter is restricted only on missing data handling technique. Data is presented below.

11.5   Different Package for Missing Data with R

11.5.1   BMTAR

This package is used for Bayesian approach for multivariate threshold autoregressive (MTAR) models with missing data using Markov chain Monte Carlo methods. One example is given in the following text.

Autoplot on Missing Data by BMTAR Package

```
library("ggplot2")
library("BMTAR")
data(missingest)
autoplot.regime_missing(missingest,1)
library(ggplot2)
data(datasim)
data = datasim$Sim$Zt
parameters=list(l=1,orders = list(pj = 1))
initial=mtarinipars(tsregime_obj = tsregime(data),
list_model = list(pars = parameters))
estim1=mtarns(ini_obj = initial,niter = 500,chain = TRUE)
autoplot.regime_model(estim1,2)
autoplot.regime_model(estim1,2)
autoplot.regime_model(estim1,3)
autoplot.regime_model(estim1,5)
data(datasim)
yt=datasim$Sim
Yt=yt$Yt
Zt=yt$Zt
data=tsregime(Yt,Zt)
autoplot.tsregime(data)
```

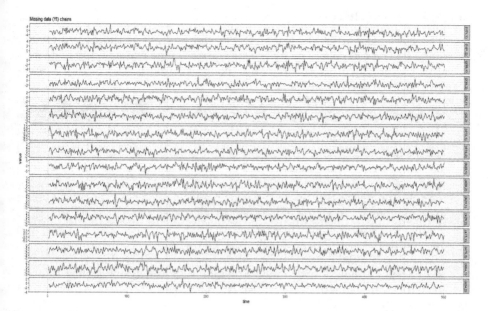

FIGURE 11.1: regime_model object ggplot for the outputs on the function outputs.

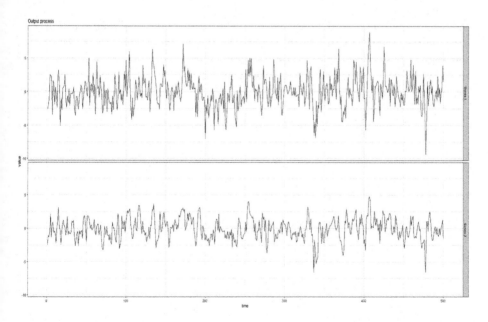

FIGURE 11.2: tsregime object ggplot for the outputs.

11.5.2   NestedCohort

The NestedCohort is dedicated for survial analysis if the covaraites are
missing. The nested cohort analysis is performed. One example to create survival plot is provided below. Secondly, the application of Cox PH by Nestec-
Cohort package is given below.

```
Survival Analysis with Missing Covariate

library("NestedCohort")
data(zinc)
mod  <-  nested.km(survfitformula="Surv(futime01,ec01==1)~ zn-
quartiles",
samplingmod="ec01×basehist",data=zinc)
plot(mod,ymin=.6,xlab="Time (Days)",ylab="Survival",
main="Survival by Quartile of Zinc",lty=1:4,)
legend(2000,0.7,c("Q1","Q2","Q3","Q4"),lty=1:4)
coxmod <- nested.coxph(coxformula="Surv(futime01,ec01==1)~
sex+agepill+smoke+drink+mildysp+moddysp+sevdysp+anyhist+
zncent",samplingmod="ec01×basehist",data=zinc)
summary(coxmod)
mod <- nested.stdsurv(outcome="Surv(futime01,ec01==1)",
exposures="znquartiles",
confounders="sex+agestr+smoke+drink+mildysp+moddysp+
sevdysp+anyhist"
samplingmod="ec01×basehist",exposureofinterest="Q4",plot=TRUE,
main="Time to Esophageal Cancer by Quartiles of Zinc",data=zinc)
```

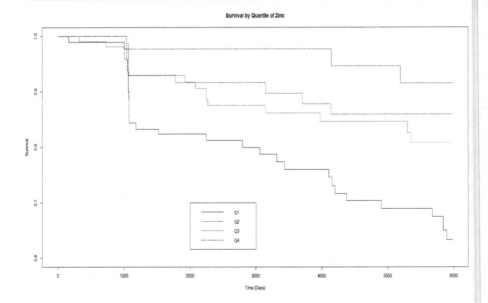

FIGURE 11.3: Survival plot by NestedCohort package.

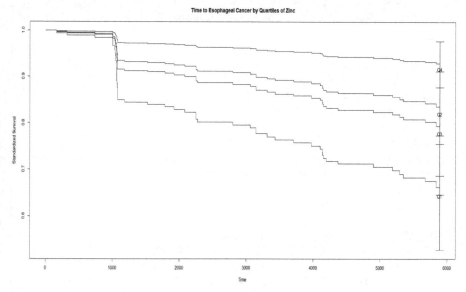

FIGURE 11.4: Standarized survival plot.

Prepare Dataset

```
  Measurment on pain score for first Arm for 14 patients at
four vistis are obtained as
Painscore1<-c(13.18,17.32,29.55,34.53,27.46,15.63,NA,NA,
39.10,20.98,9.62,29.44,20.75,30.74,23.24,34.17,
16.90,24.23,NA,NA,18.62,25.08,16.80,17.73,
15.59,21.12,NA,NA,27.95,13.01,27.19,34.90,
12.98,15.71,NA,NA,36.75,15.31,16.35,21.38,
28.60,30.38,33.50,31.80,28.68,29.28,NA,NA,
22.60,12.62,15.89,19.03,25.17,22.21,NA,NA)
visit<-c(1,1,1,1,1,1,1,1,1,1,1,1,1,1,1,
2,2,2,2,2,2,2,2,2,2,2,2,2,2,2,3,3,3,3,3,3,
3,3,3,3,3,3,3,3,3,4,4,4,4,4,4,4,4,4,4,4,4,4,4)
Similarly, for second arm is presented as
Painscore2<-c(13.18,17.32,29.55,34.53,27.46,15.63,NA,NA,
39.10,20.98,9.62,29.44,20.75,30.74,23.24,34.17,
16.90,24.23,NA,NA,18.62,25.08,16.80,17.73,
15.59,21.12,NA,NA,27.95,13.01,27.19,34.90,
12.98,15.71,NA,NA,36.75,15.31,16.35,21.38,
28.60,30.38,33.50,31.80,28.68,29.28,NA,NA,
22.60,12.62,15.89,19.03,25.17,22.21,NA,NA)
visit<-c(1,1,1,1,1,1,1,1,1,1,1,1,1,1,1,
2,2,2,2,2,2,2,2,2,2,2,2,2,2,2,3,3,3,3,3,3,
3,3,3,3,3,3,3,3,3,4,4,4,4,4,4,4,4,4,4,4,4,4,4)
```

```
Phase I Dose-Escalation Method Using OpenBUG 1

model;
{
beta1 ~ dnorm(0.0, 0.001)
beta2 ~ dnorm(0.0, 0.001)
for(i in 1:N)for (j in 2:M)Y[i,j]~ dnorm(m[i,j],T)
for(i in 1:N)for (j in 2:M)m[i,j]<-beta1 ×(1-rho)
+beta2×(visit[j]+rho×Y[i,j-1]-rho×visit[j-1])
for(i in 1:N)Y[i,1]~ dnorm(mu[i,1],T)
rho ~ dbeta(1,1)
for(i in 1:N)mu[i,1]<-beta1+beta2×visit[1]
sigma<-1/T
T ~ dgamma(.01,.01)
}
list(N = 14,M= 4,Y = structure(.Data = c(
13.18,17.32,29.55,34.53,27.46,15.63,NA,NA,39.10,20.98,
9.62,29.44,20.75,30.74,23.24,34.17,16.90,24.23,NA,NA,
18.62,25.08,16.80,17.73,15.59,21.12,NA,NA,27.95,13.01,
27.19,34.90,12.98,15.71,NA,NA,36.75,15.31,16.35,21.38,
28.60,30.38,33.50,31.80,28.68,29.28,NA,NA,22.60,12.62,
15.89,19.03,25.17,22.21,NA,NA),. Dim = c(14,4)),
visit = c(1,2,3,4))
# initial values
list(beta1 = 0,beta2 = 0,rho =.5,T= 1)
```

Similarly, code can be performed for arm two.

```
Phase I Dose-Escalation Method Using OpenBUG 2

model;
{
beta1 ~ dnorm(0.0, 0.001)
beta2 ~ dnorm(0.0, 0.001)
for(i in 1:N1){for (j in 2:M1){Y[i,j]~dnorm(mu[i,j],tau)}}
for(i in 1:N1){for (j in 2:M1){mu[i,j]<-beta1*(1-rho)
+beta2*(age[j]-rho*age[j-1])+rho*Y[i,j-1]}}
for(i in 1:N1)Y[i,1]{dnorm(mu[i,1],tau)}
rho ~ dbeta(1,1)
for(i in 1:N1){mu[i,1]<-beta1+beta2*age[1]}
tau ~ dgamma(.01,.01)
sigma<-1/tau
}
list(N1 = 17,M1 =4,Y = structure(.Data = c(10.18,14.32,26.55,31.53,
24.46,NA,23.45,11.62,
36.10,NA,6.62,26.44,
17.75,27.74,20.24,31.17,
13.90,21.23,NA,24.03,
15.62,22.08,13.80,14.73,
12.59,NA,10.63,30.99,
24.95,10.01,24.19,31.90,
9.98,NA,20.14,18.09,
33.75,12.31,13.35,18.38,
25.60,NA,NA,28.80,
25.68,26.28,15.75,21.31,
19.60,9.62,12.89,16.03,
22.17,NA,NA,NA,
24.61,22.87,17.00,17.87,
36.14,24.20,26.92,24.21,
16.85,16.43,22.93,41.27),.Dim = c(17,4)),
age = c(2,4,14,16))
# initial values
list(beta1 = 0,beta2 = 0,rho =.5,tau = 1)
```

11.6 Conclusion

Repeatedly measured immune response and QOL is typical in oncology research. Longitudinal modeling is required in repeatedly measured oncology research. The challenge of longitudinal modeling is the presence of missing data. Unfortunately, the presence of missing observation in response and covariates are frequent. Different missing value techniques are presented through MCAR, NMAR, and MAR. The MAR is presented; the likelihood function is explored. Finally, the missing values imputed. The Bayesian inference is applied, and the posterior estimate is obtained the Bayesian works through a combination of likelihood, prior and posterior estimates. The posterior estimate is presented in Table 11.1. The estimates of the posterior mean, standard deviation, and 95% credible intervals are presented in Table 11.1.

TABLE 11.1: Posterior estimate in presence of missing data

Intercept	Posterior Mean	SD	MC Error	2.5%	Median	97.5%
β_1	19.61	7.16	0.57	0.68	21.7	26.58
β_2	1.56	2.11	0.171	-0.15	0.86	8.07
rho	0.16	0.13	0.00	0.00	0.14	0.47
T	0.01	0.00	0.00	0.00	0.01	0.025

Chapter 12

Joint Longitudinal and Survival Analysis

Abstract

This chapter is dedicated about joint modeling toward analyzing the joint modeling approach. It is possible to work separately for longitudinal data and survival data. However, we will explore the joint model to handle both types of data. The Cox PH hazard model is capable of working with survival data. However, we can extend to incorporate time-dependent variables. The work is about extending the longitudinal measurement as a time-dependent covariate. A conventional approach like partial likelihood is not suitable enough in this context. Joint modeling is attempted to estimate the same parameters present in the two or more models.

12.1 Introduction

The survival outcomes are handled by the Cox model. Similarly, the linear mixed effect model is suitable to work with longitudinal measurements. The joint model plays the role of longitudinal covariate and survival outcomes. Present relation between survival and longitudinal model can be worked in two ways one by using trajectory obtained from the longitudinal observations in the hazard function of the death event. The shared random effects are also useful in this context [59]. Models can be estimated by the likelihood or Bayesian method. R packages to fit joint models are joinR, JMbayes, JM [60, 61, 62, 63, 64]. The Joint modeling was first considered in AIDS research [65, 66]. The primary interest was about survival analysis in the presence of time-dependent covariates. It was measured repeatedly with measurement error. However, drop out presence is obvious [67, 68]. Joint modeling provides less bias and more efficient estimates of the treatment effect. It is considered as most power treatment comparison method [67].

The joint model through consideration of dropout is presented as

$$p(y_i^0, d_i | x_i, z_i, w_i, \theta, \Psi) = \int \int p(y_i | x_i z_i, \theta, b_i) p(d_i | w_i, \Psi, b_i) dy_i^m db_i$$

$$= \int \int p(y_i | x_i z_i, \theta, b_i) \quad (12.1)$$

$$= \int p(y_i^0 | x_i, z_i, \theta, b_i) p(d_i | w_i, \Psi, b_i) db_i$$

The term d_i shows the time of dropout, e.g., $d_i = 3$ as $r_i = (1, 1, 0, 0, ...)$. The separate model for longitudinal data works with mixed effect model. The time-to-event model works for survival data. In time-dependent survival model, the time-dependent covariates are external because the value of the covariate at point t is not affected by the occurrence of an event at any time point $u, t > u$. Perhaps, it is not same in longitudinal setup. It is inherited property by the subject those are involved in the failure process. Therefore, the joint model is required to perform. Different software is capable of working with longitudinal and survival model separately. These are available for several years. For example, most advanced statistical software in R (R Development Core Team 2019) several packages are available to work with mixed effect modeling. Packages are nlme [69] and package lme4 [70]. Survival analysis packages are available as survival [71]. Finally, the packages available for joint modeling as well. In this work, we explored the Bayesian counterpart of the joint model through OpenBUGS.

12.2   Data Methodology

Dataset is obtained from: Gene Expression Omnibus (GEO) database (https://www.ncbi.nlm.nih.gov.in/geo/). The data accession number is GSE 65622.This illustration is obtained from a published dataset. Initially, it was published in April 2016 and thereafter in August 2016. All patients were treated with neoadjuvant chemotherapy (NACT) and followed by chemoradio-therapy (CRT). Treated patients were evaluated after four weeks after CRT completion. A total of 80 patients was considered for this analysis. Serum values were collected at baseline(visit=1), at post-NACT(visit=2), end of CRT(visit=3), post-CRT (visit=4), and at post-CRT(visit=5). The anti-body was obtained by AHH-BLG-1; RayBiotech Inc. A total of 507 proteins were measured. However, in this work, a total of 4 protein value were considered at different visits. Different gene filtration technique is performed to obtain a total of 4 protein. In addition, the value of time-to-event, i.e., death and duration of survival, is defined under the survival analysis context. The objective of this study is to obtain the effect of proteins according to their effect on cancer progression.

Now a separate discussion of survival and longitudinal is given below.

12.3 The Longitudinal Model

Suppose the longitudinal model is defined as

$$y_{ij}|\mu_{ij} \sim N(\mu_{ij}, \sigma^2) \tag{12.2}$$

and

$$\mu_{ij}\beta = x_{ij}^T\beta + z_{ij}^Tb_i \tag{12.3}$$

The times of observation for the ith individual is presented as s_{ij}. It is defined as

$$x_{ij}^T\beta = \beta_{10} + \beta_{11}s_{ij} + \beta_{12}s_{ij} \times \text{drug}_i + \beta_{13}\text{gender}_i + \beta_{14}\text{prev}_i + \beta_{15}\text{stratum}_i \tag{12.4}$$

$$z_{ij}^Tb_i = W_{1i}(s_{ij}) \tag{12.5}$$

It is formaulated as

$$W_{1i}(s_{ij}) = b_{0i} + b_{1i}s_{ij} \tag{12.6}$$

Now there is two component. One is random effect and another is random slop for time. It is presented with bivariate normal prior distribution of covariance G, i.e., $b_i \sim N(0, G)$. The noninformative prior is considered with multivariate normal distribution formation. The inverse gamma distribution is defined for $\sigma^2 \sim \text{IG}(0.1, 0.1)$. There could be a different prior choice of the inverse gamma distribution.

12.4 The Survival Model

Suppose the baseline distribution about the occurrence of death is general Weibull distribution. The duration of the interval is defined as t_i inline with the Cox proportional hazard model. Now Weibull distribution can be formulated with two parameters by scale ϕ and mean level Ψ parameter as ,

$$t_i \sim \text{Weibull}(\phi, \Psi_i) \tag{12.7}$$

Now $\phi = 1$ follows the exponential model with constand hazard model in followup period. It can be specified as

$$\log(\Psi) \sim \text{Weibull}(\phi, \Psi_i) \tag{12.8}$$

The linear predictor is formulated as

$$x_{2i}^T\beta_2 = \beta_{20} + \beta_{21}\text{drug}_i + \beta_{22}\text{gender}_i + \beta_{23}\text{prev} + \beta_{24}\text{stratum}_i \tag{12.9}$$

Finally, the random effect is formualted as

$$W_{2i} = \gamma_0 b_{0i} + \gamma_1 b_{1i} \qquad (12.10)$$

Regression parameters are assumed to have non-informative prior. Weibull parameter ϕ is defined as Gamma(1,1) prior.

12.5   The Joint Model

The objective of the joint model is to link between two models. The first step includes all similar variable in both the model. Both survival and protein value is related to treatment, trgscore ,crcargrade, tstage and yptstage. Next step is to define the common variable into the random effect term. It is assumed that b_{0i} and b_{1i} appears in both the model. The scaled parameter in the survival model is defined as γ_0 and γ_1.

12.6   Submodels Specification

Suppose T_i is defined as observed survival time for the ith subject ($i = 1, ..., n$). The minimum value between T_i and censoring time C_i. Now $T_i = \min(T_i^*, C_i)$.

$$\delta_i = I(T_i^* \leq C_i), \text{ where } I() \qquad (12.11)$$

Now $I()$ is the indicator function. It is 1 if $T_i^* \leq C_i$ and 0 otherwise. Data measured toward a time-to-event outcome is generated as $\{(T_i \delta_i), i = 1, ...n\}$. Now the longitudinal response is presented as $y_i(t)$ for the ith subject t time point measurement. Suppose the longitudinal data defined as

$$y_{ij} = \{y_i(t_{ij}), j = 1, ..., n_i\} \qquad (12.12)$$

The objective is to link the true and unobserved value of longitudinal data at time point t. The unobserved value is defined as $M_i(t)$ with the outcome event T_i^*.

$$h_i(t|M_i(t), w_i) = \lim_{dt \to 0} \Pr\{t \leq T_i^* < t + dt | T_i^* \geq t, M_i(t), w_i\}/dt \qquad (12.13)$$

$$h_i(t|M_i(t), w_i) = h_0(t)\exp\{\gamma^T w_i + \alpha m_i(t)\} \qquad (12.14)$$

Now $m_I(t) = \{M_I(U), 0 \leq U < T\}$. The history of the true unobserved longitudinal process till the observation t, is defined as $h_0()$. The term $h_0()$ is considered as baseline risk function. Now the vector of baseline covariate

TABLE 12.1: Estimates obtained through survival package in R on survival outcome

	n	Events	Median	0.95LCL	0.95UCL
Trgscore=1	32	3	NA	2668	NA
Trgscore=2	148	18	NA	1445	NA
	coef	exp(coef)	se(coef)	z	p-value
Trgscore	0.4705	1.6008	0.6267	0.751	0.453

is presented by w_i. The corresponding regression coefficients are γ. Now the parameter α is used to define the longitudinal toward the risk of death. It is required to incorporate the time-dependent covariates Suppose s_0 define the absolute continuous baseline survival function. It is defined as

$$\left\{ \int_0^{T^*} \exp\{\gamma^T \omega + \alpha m(s)\} ds \right\} \sim S_0 \tag{12.15}$$

It can be expressed as

$$h_i(t|M_i(t), \omega_i) = h_0\{V_i(t)\} + \alpha m_i(s)\}, \tag{12.16}$$

and

$$V_i(t) = \int_0^t \exp\{\gamma^T \omega_i + \alpha m_i(s)\} ds \tag{12.17}$$

Further, the baseline hazard rate can be formulated as $h_0(.)$ with a specific distribution. Now the entire covariate history is defined as $M_i(t)$ to influence the subject-specific risk factor. Now $h_0()$ can be evaluated as a subject-specific risk by $V_i(t)$). Covriate infulence $M_i(t)$ can be formualted as $S_i\{t|M_i(t)\} = S_0 V_i(t)$. Thereafter the survival models presented as $m_i(t)$ to define the value of longitudinal covariate at single time point t. But the longitudinal information is collected repeatedly and covariate or risk developed by longitudinal trajectory $M_i(t)$ as

$$y_{ij} = \{y_i(t_{ij}), j = 1, ..., n_i \tag{12.18}$$

$$y_i(t) = m_i(t) + \epsilon_i(t)$$
$$= x_i^T(t)\beta + z_i^T(t)b_i + \epsilon_i(t), \epsilon_i(t) \sim N(0, \sigma^2) \tag{12.19}$$

The fixed effect parameter presented by β. Now the random effect is $x_i(t)$[72, 73].

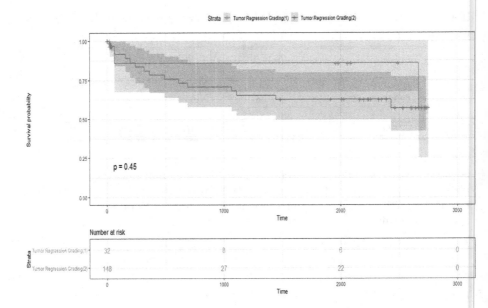

FIGURE 12.1: Kaplan-Meier curve on Tumor Regression Grading.

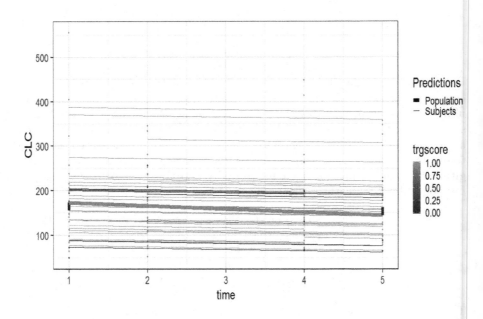

FIGURE 12.2: Linear mixed effect plot on CLC on Tumor Regression Grading.

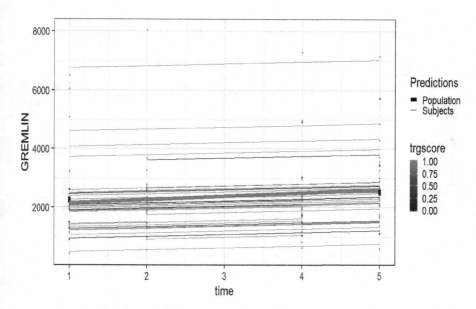

FIGURE 12.3: Linear mixed effect plot on GREMLIN on Tumor Regression Grading.

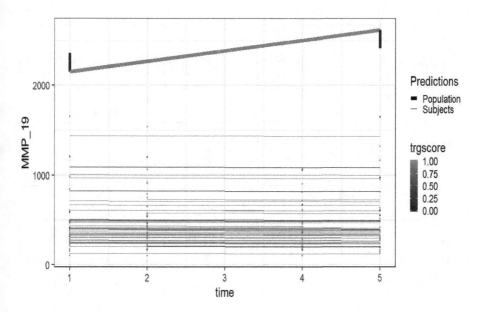

FIGURE 12.4: Linear mixed effect plot on MMP19 on Tumor Regression Grading.

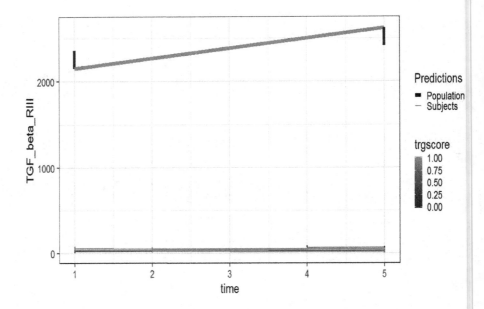

FIGURE 12.5: Linear mixed effect plot on TGFbetaRIII on Tumor Regression Grading.

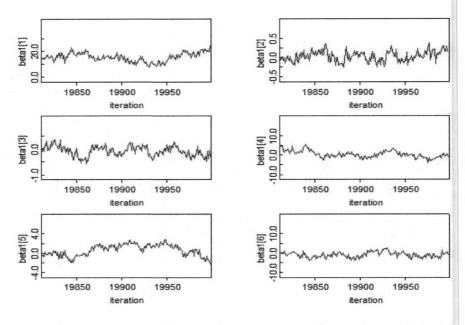

FIGURE 12.6: Traceplots on 20,000 iterations on β_1.

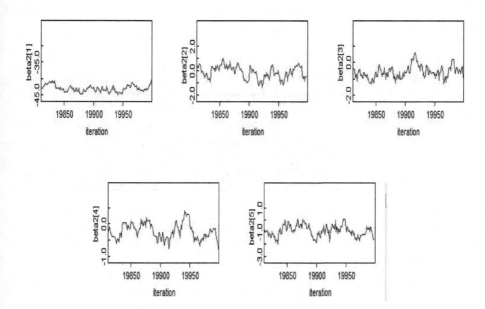

FIGURE 12.7: Traceplots on 20,000 iterations on β_2.

TABLE 12.2: Estimates obtained through nlme package in R

Outcome	Parameter	Value	Std.Error	DF	t-value	p-value
CLC	Intercept	136.27	58.54	81	2.32	0.02
	Trgscore	20.17	31.26	41	0.64	0.52
	time	-3.05	2.32	81	-1.31	0.19
GREMLIN	Intercept	3133.90	905.92	130	3.45	0.00
	Trgscore	-450.20	483.01	43	-0.93	0.35
	time	35.10	38.70	130	0.90	0.36
MMP19	Intercept	738.42	245.00	111	3.01	0.001
	Trgscore	-149.77	129.36	39	-1.15	0.25
	time	-1.13	6.53	111	-0.17	0.86
TGFbetaRIII	Intercept	33.82	11.50	59	2.93	0.00
	Trgscore	4.05	6.08	34	0.66	0.50
	time	-0.46	0.52	59	-0.87	0.38

TABLE 12.3: Model selection criteria obtained by nlme package in R

Outcome	AIC	BIC	logLik
CLC	1363.58	1377.60	-676.79
GREMLIN	2927.24	2943.00	-1458.62
MMP19	2018.83	2033.88	-1004.41
TGFbetaRIII	727.74	740.40	-358.87

TABLE 12.4: Estimates obtained through OpenBUGS code by 20,000 iteration

Parameter	Mean	SD	95% Credible Interval	Median
β_{11}	14.16	3.33	(7.33 , 20.79)	14.15
β_{12}	0.04	0.16	(-0.27 , 0.38)	0.03
β_{13}	-0.11	0.22	(-0.59 , 0.30)	-0.10
β_{14}	0.93	1.74	(-2.62 , 4.46)	0.94
β_{15}	0.53	0.90	(-1.27 , 2.39)	0.53
β_{16}	0.54	1.89	(-3.08 , 4.47)	0.51
β_{21}	-38.18	9.42	(-49.18 , -15.14)	-40.98
β_{22}	-0.14	0.44	(-1.01 , 0.73)	-0.14
β_{23}	-0.43	0.42	(-1.27 , 0.39)	-0.44
β_{24}	-0.19	0.20	(-0.60 , 0.22)	-0.19
β_{25}	-0.82	0.48	(-1.76 , 0.13)	-0.83
tauz	0.025	0.00	(0.01 , 0.04)	0.02133
r1	-0.02	1.41	(-3.26 , 2.89)	-0.00
r2	-0.32	3.36	(-8.83 , 6.54)	-0.20

OpenBUGS Code on Joint Longitudinal and Survival Model

```
model {
for (i in 1:N) {
for (j in 1:M) {
Y[i, j] ~ dnorm(muy[i, j], tauz)
muy[i, j]<- beta1[1]+beta1[2] ×
t[j]+beta1[3] × t[j]× trgscore[i]+beta1[4]× ctcaegrade[i]
+beta1[5]× tstage[i]+beta1[6] × yptstage[i]+U[i,1]+ U[i,2] × t[j] }
for (j in 1: M) {
yp1[i,j] ~ dnorm(muy[i, j], tauz)
r12[i,j]<-Y[i,j]-yp1[i,j]
sqr1[i,j]<-r12[i,j]× r12[i,j]
}
surt[i] ~ dweib(p,mut[i]) I(surt.cen[i],)
log(mut[i])<-beta2[1]+beta2[2]*trgscore[i]+
beta2[3]× ctcaegrade[i]+beta2[4]× tstage[i]+
beta2[5]× yptstage[i]+r1*U[i,1]+r2 × U[i, 2]
U[i,1:2] ~ dmnorm(U0[],tau[,])
surP[i] ~ dweib(p,mut[i]) I(surt.cen[i],)
surR[i]<-surt[i]-surP[i]
sqr2[i]<-surR[i]× surR[i]
}
mspe1<-mean(sqr1[,])
mspe2<-mean(sqr2[])
p ~ dgamma(1,1) # p <- 1
sigmaz<-1/tauz
tau[1:2,1:2]<-inverse(sigma[,])
sigmab1 ~ dunif(0,100) # priors
sigmab2 ~ dunif(0,100)
cor ~ dunif(-1,1)
sigma[1,1] <- pow(sigmab1,2)
sigma[2,2] <- pow(sigmab2,2)
sigma[1,2] <- cor ×sigmab1* sigmab2
sigma[2,1] <- sigma[1,2]
beta1[1:6] ~ dmnorm(betamu1[],Sigma1[,])
tauz ~ dgamma(0.1, 0.1)
beta2[1:5] ~ dmnorm(betamu2[],Sigma2[,])
r1 ~ dnorm(0, 0.01)
r2 ~ dnorm(0, 0.01)
```

#Importing Data

```
list(N=45,M=4,betamu1=c(0,0,0,0,0,0),
betamu2=c(0,0,0,0,0),Sigma1=structure(.Data=
c(0.01,0,0,0,0,0,0,0,0.01,0,0,0,0,0,0,0,0.01,0,0,0,0,0,0,0,
0.01,0,0,0,0,0,0,0,0.01,0,0,0,0,0,0,0,0.01),.Dim=c(6,6)),
Sigma2=structure(.Data=c(0.01,0,0,0,0,0,0,0.01,0,0,0,
0,0,0.01,0,0,0,0,0,0.01,0,0,0,0,0,0.01),.Dim=c(5,5)),
U0=c(0,0),R=structure(.Data=c(100, 0, 0, 100),
.Dim=c(2,2)),t=c(0,2,6,12),Y=structure
(.Data=c(17.53,25.60,19.85,17.82,25.68,17.23,25.30,
18.30,16.26,18.01,19.47,19.98,18.00,15.96,12.57,20.46,
19.68,13.23,12.93,8.49,8.19,7.03,8.14,7.84,14.67,17.61,
17.31,15.30,6.422,5.22,6.51,7.85,7.55,4.55,13.89,13.59,
15.00,18.34,19.95,18.92,14.81,16.40,16.10,12.77,8.32,
8.02,6.82,6.52,18.62,10.67,10.37,14.46,12.97,13.81,
12.98,10.18,9.88,12.68,13,12.70,16.34,13.94,14.56,
14.26,9.79,11.00,9.89,9.70,40.46,40.16,41.43,32.59,
11.33,8.61,10.07,12.32,8.39,10.74,10.44,12.02,8.09,
25.24,18.73,22.05,21.75,24.94,8.75,8.28,15.90,15.60,
8.45,8.93,55.56,28.12,44.68,30.08,21.51,19.15,20.05,
29.78,31.48,34.47,28.01,34.69,15.85,17.00,16.8115.30,
15.55,16.70,16.51,18.69,8.45,7.07,15.60,12.41,11.17,
8.63,10.97,27.82,44.38,11.82,12.62,11.18,7.24,7.63,
7.257,8.23,19.38,20.87,19.83,16.70,4.85,15.00,6.63,
6.37,16.98,18.39,16.67,19.19,20.60,23.51,19.36,19.65,
13.98,12.75,13.55,9.75,17.61,20.68,6.94,22.06,7.20,
7.93,6.68,8.74,16.82,16.73,15.96,15.84,3.73,33.37,
12.31,22.89,16.37,18.89,20.30,23.21,19.94,6.77,26.25,
12.45,13.25,9.45,17.31,20.38,32.26,23.80,18.68,35.64),
.Dim=c(45,4)),surt=c(2752,NA,2731,2731,2736,2719,NA,
2695,2668,NA,2645,2611,2603,2536,2492,2467,NA,NA,2393,
NA,NA,2352,2327,2255,2240,NA,2234,2199,2164,2164,NA,NA,
2088,2059,2031,NA,2010,1982,1961,1919,NA,NA,NA,1485,NA),
surt.cen=c(0,319,0,0,0,0,19,0,0,2668,0,0,0,0,0,0,1110,
2432,0,21,493,0,0,0,0,614,0,0,0,0,1067,692,0,0,0,246,0,
0,0,0,160,200,365,0,1445),trgscore=c(0,1,1,0,1,0,0,1,0,
1,0,1,0,1,1,0,0,0,1,0,1,1,1,0,0,1,0,1,1,0,0,1,1,0,1,0,0,
1,0,1,0,0,0,1,0),ctcaegrade=c(1,1,1,0,0,0,0,0,1,1,1,1,0,
1,1,1,1,1,1,1,0,1,1,1,1,0,0,0,1,1,1,0,0,0,0,0,0,0,1,0,0,
1,0,0,0),tstage=c(4,1,2,3,1,3,2,4,1,2,4,4,4,2,1,3,3,3,2,
1,2,2,4,4,1,4,2,1,1,2,2,2,1,4,4,4,4,4,4,2,2,4,3,3,1),
yptstage=c(1,0,1,1,1,1,1,0,1,1,1,0,0,0,1,1,0,1,1,1,1,0,
0,0,1,0,0,1,1,,,1,1,1,1,0,1,1,0,0,0,1,0,0,0,1))
```

```
#Importing Prior Initial Value
```

```
list(beta1=c(0,0,0,0,0,0),
tauz=1,beta2=c(0,0,0,0,0),r1=0,r2=0,U=structure(.Data=c(0,
0,0,0,0,0,0,0,0,0,0,0,0,0,0,0,0,0,0,0,0,0,0,0,0,0,0,0,0,0,
0,0,0,0,0,0,0,0,0,0,0,0,0,0,0,0,0,0,0,0,0,0,0,0,0,0,0,0,0,
0,0,0,0,0,0,0,0,0,0,0,0,0,0,0,0,0,0,0,0,0,0,0,0,0,0,0,0,0,
0,0,0,0,0),.Dim=c(45,2)))
```

12.7 Different R Package for Joint Longitudinal Model

12.7.1 joint.Cox

This package is useful for Joint Frailty-Copula Models for Tumor Progression and Death in Meta-Analysis. It used to fit the survival data and perform dynamic prediction under joint frailty-copula models for tumor progression and death.

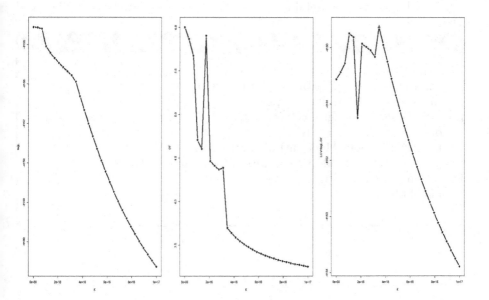

FIGURE 12.8: jointCox estimates on log-likelihood.

```
#R Code on joint.Cox Function

library("joint.Cox")
data(dataOvarian)
t.event=dataOvarian$t.event
event=dataOvarian$event
t.death=dataOvarian$t.death
death=dataOvarian$death
Z1=dataOvarian$CXCL12
group=dataOvarian$group
alpha_given=0
kappa_grid=seq(10,1e+17,length=30)
set.seed(1)
jointCox.indep.reg(t.event=t.event,event=event,
t.death=t.death,death=death,Z1=Z1,Z2=Z1,
group=group,alpha=alpha_given,kappa1=kappa_grid,
kappa2=kappa_grid,LCV.plot=TRUE,Adj=500)
```

12.7.2   JM

This JM package is useful for Joint Modeling of Longitudinal and Survival Data.

```
#R Code on JM Function

library("JM")
fitLME <- lme(log(serBilir) ~ drug × year,
random = ~ 1 | id, data = pbc2)
fitSURV <- survreg(Surv(years, status2) ~ drug,
data = pbc2.id, x = TRUE)
fitJOINT <- jointModel(fitLME, fitSURV, timeVar ="year")
plot(fitJOINT, 3, add.KM = TRUE, col ="red",lwd = 2)
par(mfrow = c(2, 2))
plot(fitJOINT)
```

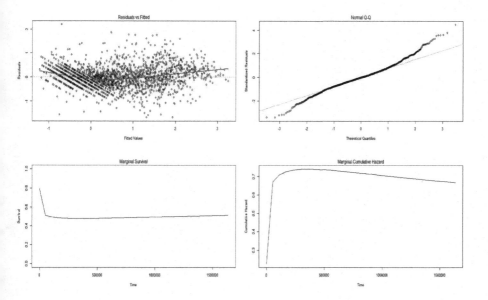

FIGURE 12.9: JM package estimate of residuals.

Chapter 13

Covariance modeling

Abstract

The mixed-effect model is useful to analyze the longitudinal data. Conventionally, the patient-specific changes are considered as random. The random effect model is supposed to perform the analysis. However, the random effect model found that the correlation between all the observations is the same. It assumed that the correlation coefficient is the same for all the patients who are the same as well. Nevertheless, these assumptions are not correct always. Correlation always depends on the time gap between the observations. It is patients specific. It is better to use a random coefficient model while the response variable is linked as the time of interest. It suits to allow the random slopes varies between the patients. Different covariance structures are detailed. Covariance structure handling techniques are illustrated with R and OpenBUG software.

13.1 Introduction

It is assumed that the patients will have different covariance, and the random effect model can not capture it. The covariance structure can be defined separately from random effects. It helps to consider the specific pattern of covariance for each visit. Sometimes, visit wise observations are considered as same for patients. Now for a clinical trial, a specific pattern across the periods could be defined same between the observations appeared on the same patients. We do define the covariance pattern by matrix R. This matrix provides that the observations are correlated. It is presented as

$$R = \begin{pmatrix} R_1 & 0 & 0 & 0 & 0 \\ 0 & R_2 & 0 & 0 & 0 \\ 0 & 0 & R_3 & 0 & 0 \\ 0 & 0 & 0 & R_4 & 0 \\ 0 & 0 & 0 & 0 & R_5 \end{pmatrix} \qquad (13.1)$$

13.2   Covariance Patterns

The mixed-effect model is suitable to work with different types of co-variance pattern. The pattern of covariance dependent on fixed times. It is easy to define the covariance pattern, while observations are equally spaced. Sometimes, the time intervals are not equal, and covariance patterns become challenging. The commercial software mixed effect modeling code can handle different types of covariance pattern. Suppose there are four-time points observations. R_i matrices define the covariance pattern. The general trend is defined as (i). The variance of the responses can be defined as σ_i^2. It may vary from time to time. With the covariance θ_{jk}, between the pair of period j and k. Now the first-order autoregressive model defined as covariance declined exponentially from time point j to k as $\theta_{jk} = \rho^{j-k}\sigma^2$. It considered that the periods are equally spaced. It defined as the 'natural' model. Sometimes, observations are not equally spaced. For example, after delivering chemotherapeutic drug patients may not be observed with equal time points. It may be required to keep them rapidly with unequal time intervals. Different types of covariance patterns are like (I) General, (II) First Order, (III) Compound symmetry, and (IV) Toeplitz.

(I) General

$$R = \begin{pmatrix} \sigma_1^2 & \theta_{12} & \theta_{13} & \theta_{14} \\ \theta_{12} & \sigma_2^2 & \theta_{23} & \theta_{24} \\ \theta_{13} & \theta_{23} & \sigma_3^2 & \theta_{34} \\ \theta_{14} & \theta_{24} & \theta_{34} & \sigma_4^2 \end{pmatrix} \tag{13.2}$$

(II) First Order

$$R = \begin{pmatrix} \sigma_1^2 & \theta_{12} & \theta_{13} & \theta_{14} \\ \theta_{12} & \sigma_2^2 & \theta_{23} & \theta_{24} \\ \theta_{13} & \theta_{23} & \sigma_3^2 & \theta_{34} \\ \theta_{14} & \theta_{24} & \theta_{34} & \sigma_4^2 \end{pmatrix} \tag{13.3}$$

(III) Compound symmetry

$$R = \begin{pmatrix} \sigma_1^2 & \theta_{12} & \theta_{13} & \theta_{14} \\ \theta_{12} & \sigma_2^2 & \theta_{23} & \theta_{24} \\ \theta_{13} & \theta_{23} & \sigma_3^2 & \theta_{34} \\ \theta_{14} & \theta_{24} & \theta_{34} & \sigma_4^2 \end{pmatrix} \tag{13.4}$$

(IV) Toeplitz

$$R = \begin{pmatrix} \sigma^2 & \theta_1 & \theta_2 & \theta_3 \\ \theta_1 & \sigma^2 & \theta_1 & \theta_2 \\ \theta_{13} & \theta_{23} & \sigma_3^2 & \theta_{34} \\ \theta_{14} & \theta_{24} & \theta_{34} & \sigma_4^2 \end{pmatrix} \tag{13.5}$$

There are two methods to handle the covariance pattern for repeatedly measure data: (I) Random effect model, (II) Multivariate normal distribution. The random effect model can address the compound symmetry pattern. However, it is required to perform the sphericity test before assuming the compound symmetry model. In case the sphericity test failed then it is necessary to achieve multivariate normal distribution. The multivariate normal distribution can consider the general covariance pattern. The multivariate normal distribution can address several covariance patterns. Perhaps, missing data inflated data can not be dealing with the multivariate normal distribution. Multiple imputation techniques are needed to overcome the missing values, and after that, covariance patterns can be taken care of suitable modeling. The suitable covariance pattern is general covariance if the measurements differ between the time points. Different variance for repeatedly measured data can be addressed by (V) Heterogeneous uncorrelated, (VI) Heterogeneous Compound Symmetry, (VII) Heterogeneous first-order autoregressive, and (VIII) Heterogeneous Toeplitz. (V) Heterogeneous uncorrelated

$$R_i = \begin{pmatrix} \sigma_1^2 & 0 & 0 & 0 \\ 0 & \sigma_2^2 & 0 & 0 \\ 0 & 0 & \sigma_3^2 & 0 \\ 0 & 0 & 0 & \sigma_4^2 \end{pmatrix} \tag{13.6}$$

(VI)Heterogeneous Compound Symmetry.

$$R_i = \begin{pmatrix} \sigma_1^2 & \rho\sigma_1\sigma_2 & \rho^2\sigma_1\sigma_3 & \rho^3\sigma_1\sigma_4 \\ \rho\sigma_1\sigma_2 & \sigma_2^2 & \rho\sigma_2\sigma_3 & \rho^2\sigma_2\sigma_4 \\ \rho^2\sigma_1\sigma_3 & \rho\sigma_2\sigma_3 & \sigma_3^2 & \rho\sigma_3\sigma_4 \\ \rho\sigma_1\sigma_4 & \rho^2\sigma_2\sigma_4 & \rho\sigma_3\sigma_4 & \sigma_4^2 \end{pmatrix} \tag{13.7}$$

(VII) Heterogeneous First-Order Autoregressive.

$$R_i = \begin{pmatrix} \sigma_1^2 & \rho\sigma_1\sigma_2 & \rho^2\sigma_1\sigma_3 & \rho^3\sigma_1\sigma_4 \\ \rho\sigma_1\sigma_2 & \sigma_2^2 & \rho^2\sigma_2\sigma_3 & \rho^2\sigma_2\sigma_4 \\ \rho^2\sigma_1\sigma_3 & \rho\sigma_2\sigma_3 & \sigma_3^2 & \rho\sigma_3\sigma_4 \\ \rho^3\sigma_1\sigma_4 & \rho^2\sigma_2\sigma_4 & \rho_1\sigma_3\sigma_4 & \sigma_4^2 \end{pmatrix} \tag{13.8}$$

(VIII) Heterogeneous Toeplitz

$$R_i = \begin{pmatrix} \sigma_1^2 & \rho_1\sigma_1\sigma_2 & \rho_2\sigma_1\sigma_3 & \rho_3\sigma_1\sigma_4 \\ \rho_1\sigma_1\sigma_2 & \sigma_2^2 & \rho_1\sigma_2\sigma_3 & \rho_2\sigma_2\sigma_4 \\ \rho_2\sigma_1\sigma_3 & \rho_1\sigma_2\sigma_3 & \sigma_3^2 & \rho_1\sigma_3\sigma_4 \\ \rho_3\sigma_1\sigma_4 & \rho_2\sigma_2\sigma_4 & \rho_1\sigma_3\sigma_4 & \sigma_4^2 \end{pmatrix} \tag{13.9}$$

The covariance structure sometimes changes differently between the therapeutic arms. It may be possible that the measurements are more correlated among arm A than arm B. The covariance matrix formulated as

$$R = \begin{pmatrix} \sigma_A^2 & \theta_A & \theta_A & 0 & 0 & 0 & 0 & 0 & 0 \\ \theta_A & \sigma_A^2 & \theta_A & 0 & 0 & 0 & 0 & 0 & 0 \\ \theta_A & \theta_A & \sigma_A^2 & 0 & 0 & 0 & 0 & 0 & 0 \\ 0 & 0 & 0 & \sigma_B^2 & \theta_B & \theta_B & 0 & 0 & 0 \\ 0 & 0 & 0 & \theta_B & \sigma_B^2 & \theta_B & 0 & 0 & 0 \\ 0 & 0 & 0 & \theta_B & \theta_B & \sigma_B^2 & 0 & 0 & 0 \\ 0 & 0 & 0 & 0 & 0 & 0 & \sigma_A^2 & \theta_A & \theta_A \\ 0 & 0 & 0 & 0 & 0 & 0 & \theta_A & \sigma_A^2 & \theta_A \\ 0 & 0 & 0 & 0 & 0 & 0 & \theta_A & \theta_A & \sigma_A^2 \end{pmatrix} \tag{13.10}$$

It may possible that the covariance pattern is negligible in nature. Some time several repeated measurements make the correlation structure poor. The R_i matrix by setting the 'band' correlation helps to work with the correlation pattern. The band with size 3 is provided below. This practice reduces the correlation parameter into minimal size.

$$R_i = \begin{pmatrix} \sigma_1^2 & \theta_{12} & \theta_{13} & 0 \\ \theta_{12} & \sigma_2^2 & \theta_{23} & \theta_{24} \\ \theta_{13} & \sigma_{23}^2 & \sigma_3^2 & \theta_{34} \\ 0 & \theta_{24} & \theta_{34} & \sigma_4^2 \end{pmatrix} \tag{13.11}$$

There are different covariance patterns available. It is difficult to choose the appropriate one. The approach is to select the most suitable one that fits with the data. It also generated with standard error with fixed effect. Sometimes the presence of more covariance parameters may increase the chance of overfitting. Likelihood testing is useful to explore the amount of overfitting. Different types of covariance patterns are available. It is not easy to select an appropriate one. It is suitable to define the best covariance by fitting the data. The standard error for the fixed effects model estimate is useful to understand the covariance pattern. The model diagnostic criteria are useful to test the best covariance structure. It is defined as

$$\text{AIC} = \log(L) - q \tag{13.12}$$

Now the covariance pattern is defined by q. Suppose the fixed effect is p represent the number of observations. The total number of observations are N. It is presented as

$$\text{SIC} = \log(L) - (q\log(N - p))/2 \tag{13.13}$$

Models presented with the lower value of AIC and SIC define as better fits. This model selection criterion is available in the R software package 'nlme'. Alternatively, the likelihood ratio test is useful to understand the covariance parameters are important or not. The likelihood ratio test of the statistics is defined as

$$2(\log(L_1) - \log(L_2)) \sim \chi_{DF}^2 \tag{13.14}$$

Now the difference in the number of covariance parameter is fitted by DF.

13.3 Covariance Patterns Challenges

It is always difficult to perform a test to understand a large covariance structure. The best step would be to start with compound symmetry or first-order autoregressive modeling. The task is to look about intricate patterns present or not. The appearance of the sophisticated design is fixed by likelihood value. However, it is possible to have a complex model while the dataset is large enough. However, large datasets always required to understand intricate covariance patterns. Now the covariance pattern is not of intrinsic interest. The compound symmetry pattern may be adequate to estimate the treatment effect and standard errors. Now model checking is required to explore the pattern. Now if the difference is small, then the compound symmetry pattern can be used with reasonable confidence.

13.4 Illustration with Protein-Gene Expression Time-Course Data

```
#Running the Function as Gamma Distribution

library("blme")
data("sleepstudy", package="lme4")
fm1<-blmer(Reaction ~ Days+(0+Days|Subject),sleepstudy,
cov.prior=gamma)
summary(fm1)
```

```
# R Output on Gamma Distribution

Cov prior   : Subject ~ gamma(shape = 2.5, rate = 0,
posterior.scale = sd, common.scale = TRUE)
Prior dev   : 3.9858

Linear mixed model fit by REML ['blmerMod']
Formula: Reaction ~ Days + (0 + Days | Subject)
   Data: sleep study

REML criterion at convergence: 1766.6

Scaled residuals:
    Min      1Q   Median      3Q     Max
-3.5411 -0.5565  0.0534  0.6239  4.6236

Random effects:
 Groups   Name Variance Std. Dev.
 Subject  Days 58.49    7.648
 Residual      833.79   28.875
Number of obs: 180, groups:  Subject, 18

Fixed effects:
            Estimate Std. Error t value
(Intercept)  251.405      4.000  62.847
Days          10.467      1.952   5.362

Correlation of Fixed Effects:
     (Intr)
Days -0.324
```

```
#Running the Function as Gamma Distribution

fm2 <- blmer(Reaction ~ Days + (0 + Days|Subject),
sleepstudy,cov.prior = gamma(shape = 2, rate = 0.5,
posterior.scale ='sd'))
summary(fm2)
```

```
# Gamma Prior with Different Rate and Scale

Cov prior  : Subject ~ gamma(shape = 2, rate = 0.5,
posterior.scale = sd, common.scale = TRUE)
Prior dev  : 5.7375

Linear mixed model fit by REML ['blmerMod']
Formula: Reaction ~ Days + (0 + Days | Subject)
   Data: sleep study

REML criterion at convergence: 1766.6

Scaled residuals:
    Min      1Q  Median      3Q     Max
-3.5281 -0.5575  0.0533  0.6242  4.6146

Random effects:
 Groups    Name Variance Std. Dev.
 Subject  Days  55.9      7.477
 Residual       837.3    28.935
Number of obs: 180, groups:  Subject, 18

Fixed effects:
            Estimate Std. Error t value
(Intercept) 251.405      4.009  62.717
Days         10.467      1.916   5.464

Correlation of Fixed Effects:
     (Intr)
Days -0.330
```

#Prior as Inverse Gamma Distribution

```
fm3 <- blmer( Reaction ~ Days + (0 + Days | Subject),
sleepstudy,cov.prior =invgamma(shape = 0, scale = 0,
posterior.scale ='sd'))
summary(fm3)
```

#Inverse Gamma Prior with Different Rate and Scale

```
Cov prior  : Subject ~ gamma(shape = 0, scale = 0,
posterior.scale = sd, common.scale = TRUE)
Prior dev  : -Inf

Linear mixed model fit by REML ['blmerMod']
Formula: Reaction ~ Days + (0 + Days | Subject)
   Data: sleep study

REML criterion at convergence: 1893.7

Scaled residuals:
    Min      1Q  Median      3Q     Max
-2.3231 -0.5760  0.0324  0.5479  2.9331

Random effects:
 Groups   Name Variance Std. Dev.
 Subject  Days 0        0.00
 Residual      2277     47.71
Number of obs: 180, groups:  Subject, 18

Fixed effects:
            Estimate Std. Error t value
(Intercept) 251.405    6.610    38.033
Days         10.467    1.238     8.454

Correlation of Fixed Effects:
     (Intr)
Days -0.843
```

```
#Prior as Wishart Distribution
```

```
fm4 <- blmer(Reaction ~ Days + (1 + Days|Subject),
sleepstudy,cov.prior = wishart)
summary(fm4)
```

```
#Wishart Prior Distributionn
```

```
Cov prior  : Subject ~ wishart(df = 4.5, scale = Inf,
posterior.scale = cov, common.scale = TRUE)
Prior dev  : 4.1552

Linear mixed model fit by REML ['blmerMod']
Formula: Reaction ~ Days + (1 + Days | Subject)
   Data: sleep study

REML criterion at convergence: 1743.8

Scaled residuals:
    Min      1Q  Median      3Q     Max
-4.0094 -0.4665  0.0167  0.4698  5.2207

Random effects:
 Groups   Name        Variance Std.Dev. Corr
 Subject  (Intercept) 646.16   25.420
          Days         40.33    6.351   0.00
 Residual             644.93   25.396
Number of obs: 180, groups:  Subject, 18

Fixed effects:
            Estimate Std. Error t value
(Intercept)  251.405      6.948   36.18
Days          10.467      1.636    6.40

Correlation of Fixed Effects:
     (Intr)
Days -0.170
```

#Prior as Invwishart Distribution

```
(fm5 <- blmer(Reaction ~ Days + (1 + Days|Subject),
sleepstudy,cov.prior = invwishart(df=
5, scale = diag(0.5, 2)))
summary(fm5)
```

#Inverse Wishart Prior Distribution

```
Cov prior  : Subject ~ invwishart(df = 5, scale = c(0.5
, 0, 0, 0.5),
posterior.scale = cov, common.scale = TRUE)
Prior dev  : 1.7533

Linear mixed model fit by REML ['blmerMod']
Formula: Reaction ~ Days + (1 + Days | Subject)
   Data: sleep study

REML criterion at convergence: 1743.7

Scaled residuals:
    Min      1Q  Median      3Q     Max
-3.9930 -0.4627  0.0128  0.4683  5.2088

Random effects:
 Groups   Name        Variance Std.Dev. Corr
 Subject  (Intercept) 634.52   25.190
          Days         38.59    6.212   0.04
 Residual             647.68   25.450
Number of obs: 180, groups:  Subject, 18

Fixed effects:
            Estimate Std. Error t value
(Intercept)  251.405      6.905  36.408
Days          10.467      1.606   6.517

Correlation of Fixed Effects:
     (Intr)
Days -0.145
```

```
#Prior as PenaltyFn

penaltyFn <- function(sigma)
dcauchy(sigma, 0, 10, log = TRUE)
fm6 <- blmer(Reaction ~ Days + (0 + Days|Subject),
sleepstudy,cov.prior = custom(penaltyFn,
chol = TRUE, scale = "log"))
summary(fm6)
```

```
# Prior as PenaltyFn

Cov prior  : Subject ~ custom(fn = penaltyFn, chol = TRUE,
scale = log, common.scale = TRUE)
Prior dev  : 6.8959

Linear mixed model fit by REML ['blmerMod']
Formula: Reaction ~ Days + (0 + Days | Subject)
   Data: sleep study

REML criterion at convergence: 1766.5

Scaled residuals:
    Min      1Q  Median      3Q     Max
-3.5104 -0.5588  0.0541  0.6244  4.6022

Random effects:
 Groups   Name Variance Std. Dev.
 Subject  Days 52.7     7.26
 Residual      842.0    29.02
Number of obs: 180, groups:  Subject, 18

Fixed effects:
            Estimate Std. Error t value
(Intercept) 251.405     4.020   62.539
Days         10.467     1.869    5.599

Correlation of Fixed Effects:
     (Intr)
Days -0.340
```

#Prior as Normal Distribution as Fixed Effect

```
fm7 <- blmer(Reaction ~ Days + (1 + Days|Subject),
sleepstudy,cov.prior = NULL,fixef.prior = normal)
summary(fm7)
```

#Normal Distribution with Fixed Effect as Prior Distribution

```
Fixef prior: normal(sd = c(10, 2.5), corr = 0,
 common.scale = TRUE)
Prior dev  : 24.0661

Linear mixed model fit by REML ['blmerMod']
Formula: Reaction ~ Days + (1 + Days | Subject)
   Data: sleep study

REML criterion at convergence: 1743.6

Scaled residuals:
    Min     1Q  Median     3Q     Max
-3.9688 -0.4628  0.0222  0.4674  5.1974

Random effects:
 Groups    Name         Variance Std.Dev. Corr
 Subject   (Intercept)  613.67   24.772
           Days          35.13    5.927   0.06
 Residual               650.42   25.503
Number of obs: 180, groups:  Subject, 18

Fixed effects:
            Estimate Std. Error t value
(Intercept)  251.229      6.822  36.825
Days          10.467      1.545   6.773

Correlation of Fixed Effects:
     (Intr)
Days -0.137
```

```
#Prior as Normal Distribution
```

```
fm8 <- blmer(Reaction ~ Days + (1 + Days|Subject),
sleepstudy,cov.prior = NULL,fixef.prior=
normal(cov = diag(0.5, 2), common.scale = FALSE))
summary(fm8)
```

```
#Normal Prior Distribution
```

```
Fixef prior: normal(sd = c(0.7071, 0.7071),
corr = 0, common.scale = FALSE)
Prior dev  : 2.2959

Linear mixed model fit by REML ['blmerMod']
Formula: Reaction ~ Days + (1 + Days | Subject)
   Data: sleep study

REML criterion at convergence: 1830.7

Scaled residuals:
    Min      1Q  Median      3Q     Max
-3.9442 -0.4592 -0.0049  0.4604  5.1673

Random effects:
 Groups   Name        Variance Std.Dev. Corr
 Subject  (Intercept) 63677.9  252.34
          Days          141.6   11.90   0.88
 Residual               655.0   25.59
Number of obs: 180, groups:  Subject, 18

Fixed effects:
            Estimate Std. Error t value
(Intercept)  0.03354    0.70696   0.047
Days         0.04581    0.64477   0.071

Correlation of Fixed Effects:
     (Intr)
Days 0.007
```

Part IV

Bayesian in Diagnostics Test Statistics

Chapter 14

Bayesian Inference in Mixed-Effect Model

Abstract

It becomes an attractive choice to get a higher blockade of cancer cell progression by Molecular Targeted Agents (MTA). The statistical methodology for MTA has required attention. The literature on early phase dose-finding studies with MTA is minimal. The dose-finding design in the MTA setting is attempted by continuously updating the influence of the biological agent. In this chapter, the Bayesian approach is presented to perform the linear mixed effect models. The model has performed with the Markov chain Monte Carlo (MCMC) method. It provides an algorithm to assign different possible doses for each subject. It helps to define the optimum treatment on MTA value. It is potent enough to accumulate the doses information by capturing their variability, an overlooked area in the conventional model. A simulation study is performed to create dose values. This work is suitable for Phase-I dose without the MTD or DLT. The intention is to look for specific biomarker value by contributing effect of different dose. The illustration in this work will help to build a dose-response curve to detect the best effective treatment through MTA in a group of patients.

14.1 Introduction

The likelihood estimation is one way to perform a linear mixed effect model. However, another alternative is Bayesian inference. Earlier, it was challenging to achieve Bayesian mixed-effect model through R. However, R with "glm" and "lmer" package becomes a useful tool to perform a mixed-effect model with R. But these two packages helpful to work with likelihood-based models. It is a fact that Bayesian is not a replacement of maximum likelihood estimation. However, Bayesian is easy to perform in recent years. It requires to the known fundamental concept of Bayesian before application. Hypothesis testing is not the same in Bayesian inference. The likelihood-based method obtained by "lme4" for the parameter θ and data y looks by Bayesian theorem

$$p(\theta|y)\propto l(\theta|y)p(\theta) \tag{14.1}$$

The term $p(\theta|y)$ used to define the posterior probability. We can only understand the parameter from the data. It can give us predictions. The prior probability is $p(\theta)$. The specification of the prior is the challenging task to explore Bayesian modeling. The conventional dose-finding trial is based on controlling the tolerable dose. Now the cytotoxic agents are tested about the maximum tolerated dose (MTD). Now it is anticipated that drug response will be higher through high doses. However, the toxicity will also increase with increased dose. Similarly, the probability of toxicity will also incline. The method used to identify the best effective dose is well known as rule-base as a 3 + 3 design. Now the model-based design can be classified as Continual Reassessment Method (CRM) [74, 75], and modified CRM [76, 77, 78], Time-to-Event CRM (TITE-CRM) [79] and Escalation with Overdose Control (EWOC) design [80]. Now the challenge is that a small sample size needs to be lesser to take any decision about drug-dose. The maximum tolerable dose that any patient can tolerate is defined as Dose Limiting Toxicity(DLT). In this continuation, it is required to promote the model-based designs [81, 82]. But making any decision about effective dose by looking MTD is not enough [83, 84, 85, 86]. The drugs or other essences promote tumor progression [87]. It becomes an attractive choice to get a higher blockade of cancer cell progression by molecular targeted agents (MTA) .The transduction pathway by the bypassing mechanism [88]. The statistical methodology for MTA is required to apply. The literature on early phase dose-finding studies with MTA is minimal. The dose-finding design in the MTA setting is attempted by continuously updating the influence of the biological agent [89]. Recently, there is an attempt to compare the dose-efficacy by curves [90]. The dose-toxicity modeling can be performed by change-point analysis [91] is performed to estimate the best effective dose in the MTA setup. Several methodologies are about balancing between dose-efficacy and dose-toxicity. However, the preliminary assumption that the increase of dose will be more efficient for treatment. Alternatively, it is also observed that increasing dose can reduce the dose efficiency [89, 91]. It is aimed to develop a novel dose-finding model of MTA. It is required to the point that best effective dose in MTA or better called the optimum biological dose (OBD). There are computationally possibilities to work with Bayesian inference by a linear mixed effect model [92, 93, 94] to get the OBD. Initial attempts motivate us to propose a model with a mixed effect model set up to deal with OBD. The dose-Response model is performed. Different dose levels are defined as covariates on treatment efficacy. The autoregressive [95] and dynamic linear mixed effect modeling [96] are considered. In contrast, a flexible-dose regime is presented to treated patients to obtain the best effective dose. The non-linear varying coefficient is considered to run the linear mixed-effect model. The best effective dose is obtained by a linear setting

[97]. Similarly, a mixed-effect model with a Gaussian process functional form is adopted. The non-parametric Gaussian process component addresses the fixed effect and parametric Gaussian as the random effect component [98]. The challenge is to link between earlier time point measurements on the current dose level. The index value can be used to model the dependence between response with time-varying predictor values [99] or by the coefficient of a regression model as time-dependent functions [100]. The functional form to serve the random effect mixed effect model is initiated [101]. The Gaussian process regression model is obtained to estimate the functional form of random effect [102, 103]. In this chapter, the Bayesian approach is presented to perform the linear mixed effect models. The model has performed with the Markov chain Monte Carlo (MCMC) method. Mixture distribution is adopted with point mass and continuous distribution to select the variables as fixed or random effects. The MCMC is used to obtain the posterior estimates. The primary aim of dose-response studies is to classify the individual level response change for different doses or agents. Based on this work we can build a dose-response curve to detect the best effective dose through MTA in a group of patients.

14.2 Likelihood Function with Doses and Measurement Process

The repeatedly measured continuous variable for each patients and corresponding dose is defined as

$$Y_{i,t}^{(h)} = (Y_{i,0}, Y_{i,1}, Y_{i,2}, ..., Y_{i,t})^T \qquad (14.2)$$

The response value measured as the vector of responses from 0 to t for the individuals ($i = 1, ..., N$). The prior to baseline measurements are defined by superscript (h) as $Y_{i,t}^{(h)}$ and baseline measurements by $Y_{i,0}$ and the k-th time point measurements are defined as $Y_{i,k}$. Further, the administered doses are defined as

$$x_{i,t}^{(d)} = (X_{i,1}, X_{i,2}, ..., X_{i,t})^T \qquad (14.3)$$

for the time point from 1 to t. The doses are defined as time dependent covariates. The doses administered between time points $t-1$ and t are defined as $X_{i,t}$. The time of the last measurement for the ith subject is defined as T_i. The likelihood function is defined as

$$L(\theta, \psi) = f(Y_{i,T_i}^{(h)}, X_{i,T_i}^{(d)} | Z_i, \theta, \psi) \qquad (14.4)$$

The parameter θ and ψ are adopted to define the measurement process and dose process, respectively. The time independent covariates are defined by Z_i, with the measurement process

$$L(\theta) = f(Y_{i,0}|Z_i, \theta) \prod_{t=1}^{T_i} f(Y_{i,t}|Y_{i,t-1}^{(h)}, X_{i,t}^{(d)}, Z_i, \theta) \qquad (14.5)$$

The likelihood for the dose process is generated as

$$L(\psi) = f(X_{i,1}|Y_{i,0}, Z_i, \psi) \prod_{t=2}^{T_i} f(X_{i,t}|Y_{i,t-1}^{(h)}, X_{i,t-1}^{(d)}, Z_i, \psi) \qquad (14.6)$$

The compact likelihood function is prepared as

$$L(\theta, \psi) = L(\theta) \times L(\psi) \qquad (14.7)$$

The factorization process is separated as $f(a, b) = f(a|b)f(b)$.

$$f(Y_{i,T_i}^{(h)}, X_{i,T_i}^{(d)}|Z_i, \theta, \psi) = f(Y_{i,0}, ..., Y_{i,T_i}, X_{i,1}, ...X_{i,T_i}|Z_i, \theta, \psi) \qquad (14.8)$$

$$f(Y_{i,T_i}^{(h)}, X_{i,T_i}^{(d)}|Z_i, \theta, \psi) = f(Y_{i,T_i}|Y_{i,T_i-1}^{(h)}, X_{i,T_i}^{(d)}, Z_i, \theta) \times f(Y_{i,T_i-1}^{(h)}, X_{i,T_i}^{(d)}|Z_i, \theta, \psi) \qquad (14.9)$$

and so on.

14.3 Linear Mixed-Effects Model

The linear mixed-effect model can jointly handle fixed and random effect models [104, 105]. Different assumptions are required. There is shallow adoption of the mixed effect model for non-availability of user-friendly software. However, it is adopted primarily by open-source software R [106, 107]. Another reason for avoiding the linear mixed-effect models is the presences of complexity in comparison to the regression models. It requires a high level of computational expertise [108]. The mathematical explanation is described below about linear mixed-effect model.

The response variable is defined with vector $Y_i = (Y_{i,0}, Y_{i,1}, Y_{i,2}, ..., Y_{i,T_i})^T$ for the i-th $(i = 1, ..., N)$ subject measured at 0 to T_i. The linear mixed effect model is defined as

$$Y_i = X_i\beta + Z_i b_i + \epsilon_i \qquad (14.10)$$

The β is a $p \times 1$ vector with unknown-fixed effect, and X_i is matrix with $(T_i + 1) \times p$ for fixed effect and b_i is a $q \times 1$ vector with unknown random-effect parameters. The term Z_i is a known, $(T_i + 1) \times q$ stands for design matrix of random effects and ϵ_i stands for random errors for the vector with time $(T_i + 1) \times 1$. It is assumed that the term ϵ_i and b_i follows the i.i.d with mean zero and covariance matrix R_i and G, respectively.

14.4 Autoregressive Linear Mixed-Effects Model

The response is free with toxicity effects. The novelty of our method is to decide the best effective dose for toxicity free OBD measurements. The parametric assumptions are not required. The auto-regressive covariance structures are defined to declare the optimum dose. The conventional method is decided based on DLT, and no patients are permitted to prescribe more than DLT once if it is archived. However, our model is free from DLT module. Best doses are decided from available all lower doses. Our proposed method provides scope about intra-patient dose reductions at any time. It is an alternative about the administration of multiple doses and therefore, the consequence of DLT [109, 110]. The autoregressive linear model in this direction is defined as

$$Y_i = \rho F_i Y_i + X_i \beta + Z_i b_i + \epsilon_i \qquad (14.11)$$

The time expresser matrix is $(T_i + 1) \times (T_i + 1)$. The elements below the diagonal are 1 and above are 0. The earlier time point response is defined as $F_i Y_i = (0, Y_{i,0}, Y_{i,1}, ..., Y_{i,T_i})^T$. The regression coefficient linked with earlier response to post responses is ρ. The unconditional response vector is defined as

$$Y_i = (I_i - \rho F_i)^{-1}(X_i \beta + Z_i b_i + \epsilon_i) \qquad (14.12)$$

Here, I_i is a $(T_i + 1) \times (T_i + 1)$ identity matrix. The linear mixed effect model extended with autoregressive model is prepared as

$$Y_i = X_i^* \beta^* + Z_i b_i + \epsilon_i \qquad (14.13)$$

where $\beta^* = (\beta^T, \rho)^T$ and $X_i^* = (X_i, F_i Y_i)$.

14.5 Linear Mixed-Effects Model Compatible with Dose Response

The mixed effect model compitable with repeatedly measured doses are defined as

$$Y_{i,t} = (\beta_{\text{int}} + b_{\text{int i}}) + (\beta_{\text{dose}} + b_{\text{dose},i})X_{i,t} + \epsilon_{i,t} \qquad (14.14)$$

The responses are measured with steady states by $Y_{i,t}$ and $X_{i,t}$ for the response levels and doses for i-th subject respectively. The fixed effect is defined as $\beta = (\beta_{\text{int}}, \beta_{dose})^T$ and the random-effects $b_i = (b_{\text{int i}}, b_{\text{dose i}})^T$ with the intercept and the dose effect. Further, it is assumed that b_i follows the normal distribution with mean zero and covariance structure G_{ss}. It is free with baseline measurement and error term is defined by $\epsilon_{i,t}$. The error term $\epsilon_{i,t}$ follows mean zero and variance σ^2.

14.6 Autoregressive Linear Mixed Effects Model Compatible with Dose Response

The autoregressive model is defined with dose modification by

$$Y_{i,t} = \beta_{\text{base}} + b_{\text{base } i} + \epsilon_{i,t}(t = 0) \tag{14.15}$$

$$Y_{i,t} = \rho Y_{i,t-1} + (\beta_{\text{int}} + b_{\text{int } i}) + (\beta_{\text{dose}} + b_{\text{dose } i})X_{i,t} + \epsilon_{i,t} - \rho\epsilon_{i,t-1}(t > 0) \tag{14.16}$$

The term $Y_{i,t}$ and $X_{i,t}$ are the representative of response and dose contribution for the i-th subject at time point t, respectively. The fixed-effect determined by $\beta = (\beta_{base}, \beta_{int}, \beta_{dose})^T$ and random-effects by $b_i = (b_{\text{base } i}, b_{\text{int } i}, b_{\text{dose } i})^T$ for the baseline, follow-up intercept, and follow-up dose effect, respectively. It is assumed that the random-effect, i.e., b_i, follows the normal distribution with mean zero and covariance structure, i.e., unstructured as G. The assumption of ϵ_i considered as $N(0, \sigma^2)$. The autoregressive error is captured through ϵ_i. Further, the marginal representation of model for $(t > 0)$ is represented as

$$Y_{i,t} = \rho^t(\beta_{\text{base}} + b_{\text{base i}} + \sum_{j=1}^{t} \rho^{t-j}\{(\beta_{\text{int}} + b_{\text{int i}}) + (\beta_{\text{dose}} + b_{\text{dose i}})X_{i,j} + \epsilon_{i,j}\} \tag{14.17}$$

The dose effect at time point s on the response at time $t(t \geq s)$ is defined as $\rho^{t-s}(\beta_{dose} + b_{dose\ i})X_{i,s}$. It will decline while the time progressed. However, if the dose X provided repeatedly with time, then the asymptotes for the population mean and the ith subject is defined as $(1 - \rho)^{-1}(\beta_{int} + \beta_{dose}X)$ and $(1 - \rho)^{-1}(\beta_{int} + \beta_{dose} + (\beta_{dose}X + b_{dosei}X)$ respectively.

14.7 Generating Data

There is no consensus on the most appropriate methodology on MTA response for Metronomic Chemotherapy(MC). Therefore, a simulation study was performed to assess the OBD about the performance of an MC. Datasets were generated to resemble the skewed distributions seen in a motivating example. The results obtained through the linear mixed effect model and autoregressive models are given in Table 14.2 and Table 14.3, respectively. A total of 25 patients with different doses of treatments are presented. All of the patients were exposed to four different visits to measure their MTA value. The doses selected as Dose=15 mg/m^2, Dose=12.5 mg/m^2, Dose=10 mg/m^2, Dose=7.5 mg/m^2 and Dose=5 mg/m^2 respectively. The simulation techniques were performed. Dose-effect relations are established by the MCMC iterations. Two OpenBUGS programs were written for the linear mixed effect model and autoregressive effect separately. A total of 20,000 iterations were used to generate convergence statistics. The credible intervals were given in Table 14.2 and Table 14.4, respectively.

TABLE 14.1: Different doses and corresponding mean(sd) MTA response observed through simulated data.

Dose	Time1	Time2	Time3	Time4
15 mg/m^2	9.60(3.08)	9.11(1.40)	8.28(1.36)	10.47(1.22)
12.5 mg/m^2	15.65(1.69)	14.24(2.21)	14.90(1.68)	16.15(0.51)
10 mg/m^2	19.35(2.70)	19.42(1.43)	20.03(1.55)	19.38(3.23)
7.5 mg/m^2	13.37(2.09)	14.24(2.73)	14.07(1.45)	15.38(2.87)
5 mg/m^2	10.79(1.71)	9.03(1.82)	10.24(1.57)	9.59(1.53)

TABLE 14.2: Posterior estimates generated through different models through linear mixed-effect model on MTA response.

Doses	Parameter	Posterior Mean(SD)	95% HPD
15 mg/m^2	β_1 (Intercept)	9.36(0.81)	(7.81,10.93)
	β_2	0.72(0.51)	(-0.30,1.708)
	σ_1^2	0.85(2.31)	(0.13,3.50)
12.5 mg/m^2	β_3(Intercept)	14.91(0.79)	(13.34,16.45)
	β_4	-0.046(0.52)	(-1.10,1.00)
	σ_2^2	0.67(0.97)	(0.12,2.60)
10mg/m^2	β_5(Intercept)	20.47(0.84)	(18.90,22.07)
	β_6	-0.43(0.52)	(-1.40,0.55)
	σ_3^2	0.82(1.39)	(0.13,3.48)
7.5 mg/m^2	β_7(Intercept)	14.30(0.84)	(12.76,15.85)
	β_8	0.0912(0.51)	(-0.91,1.10)
	σ_4^2	0.79(1.08)	(0.14,2.99)
5 mg/m^2	β_9(Intercept)	11.23(0.79)	(9.66,12.81)
	β_{10}	-0.76(0.52)	(-1.77,0.22)
	σ_5^2	0.89(3.21)	(0.13,3.39)

TABLE 14.3: Model selection criteria of the linear mixed-effect model.

Doses	$\bar{D}$	$\hat{D}$	DIC	pD
15 mg/m^2	83.14	77.84	88.45	5.301
12.5 mg/m^2	82.96	77.5	88.41	5.451
10mg/m^2	72.86	67.45	78.27	5.408
7.5 mg/m^2	81.17	75.69	86.65	5.48
5 mg/m^2	83.06	77.74	88.37	5.311

TABLE 14.4: Posterior estimates generated through different models through autoregressive model on MTA response.

Doses	Parameter	Posterior Mean(SD)	95% HPD
15 mg/m^2	β_1 (Intercept)	4.84(6.48)	(-9.98,10.96)
	β_2	1.70(1.76)	(-0.13,5.96)
	σ_6^2	5.60(2.52)	(2.57,11.99)
12.5 mg/m^2	β_3(Intercept)	9.65(23.48)	(-35.53,52)
	β_4	4.81(23.47)	(-37.62,50)
	σ_7^2	2.06(4.80)	(0.36,8.50)
10mg/m^2	β_5(Intercept)	19.73(6.38)	(3.46,26.87)
	β_6	-1.72(1.86)	(-3.97,3.59)
	σ_8^2	46.89(27.91)	(11.84,114)
7.5 mg/m^2	β_7(Intercept)	11.87(4.30)	(0.00,16.62)
	β_8	0.60(1.12)	(-0.85,3.81)
	σ_9^2	6.12(5.71)	(2.158,23.92)
5 mg/m^2	β_9(Intercept)	11.26(2.86)	(3.42,14.83)
	β_{10}	-0.52(0.90)	(-1.73,1.88)
	σ_{10}^2	26.25(30.38)	(2.66,101.6)

14.8   Computation Support

This work is illustrated on MTA measurements. MTA measured as gene expressions occurred to measured as high-dimensional data. So it is better to present any statistical methods that can be handled with the high-dimensional setup as well. The computational flexibility toward high-dimensional data analysis is limited. Markov chain Monte Carlo (MCMC) algorithms allow computation flexibility to perform the linear mixed model [111]. There are several attempts in last two decades to computationally enrich the power of computation. There are dedicated software like MCMCglmm [112, 113, 114, 115], WinBUGS [116, 117]. However, the challenges faced by slow convergence in high-dimensional correlated data [114, 118]). The conjugate priors are only

TABLE 14.5: Model selection criteria of the autoregressive model on MTA response.

Doses	$\bar{D}$	$\hat{D}$	DIC	pD
15 mg/m^2	85.7	83.68	87.73	2.02
12.5 mg/m^2	93.75	91.45	96.05	2.29
10mg/m^2	20.78	20.25	21.31	0.53
7.5 mg/m^2	83.28	81.13	85.42	2.14
5 mg/m^2	84.67	83.39	85.94	1.27

available for Gibbs sampling to the likelihood of a parameter [114]. It is easy to work Stan software by Hamiltonian Monte Carlo simulation [118, 119]. It converges very fast, particularly for high-dimensional data [120]. The computational flexibility is obtained by collectively working with R, OpenBUGS and Stan [113]. There are dedicated available packages like "brms" and "blme" in R.

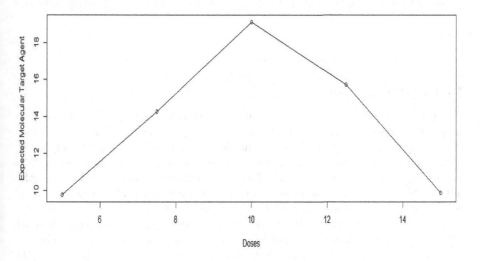

FIGURE 14.1: OBD achieved through different dose labels.

14.9   Power Analysis of the Performed Models

If a study is underpowered, then there is a possibility about the waste of resources and the real effects may not be generated [110, 121]. Similarly, a large study comes with overpowered and expensive than a real requirement [122]. A sample size calculation is required to fulfil the research queries. There are several dedicated packages those available with R to work with mixed effect model and power analysis [123, 124, 125]). There is also the provision to perform with power analysis of mixed effect by specifying the fixed and random effect component [122]. The power analysis is obtained by "SIMR" and "LME4" packages [106]. A total of 5 different doses were selected to generate the simulated data. The doses were $15mg/m^2$, $12.5mg/m^2$, $15mg/m^2$, $10mg/m^2$, $7.5mg/m^2$ and $5mg/m^2$ respectively.The MTA value as a continuous variable for 25 patients was generated, with 4-time points/visits. The MTA was assumed to follow the normal distribution with mean ten and standard deviation 2. The age interval was obtained from 21 to 45 years. The power analysis was performed with "powers" function available in SIMR package with R. A total of 10 times simulations were carried out to obtain the result. A 95% confidence interval provides the power of predictor with 65%[50.32%, 80.85%] range. The power of a selected linear mixed effect model is relatively robust.

14.10   Discussion

Our proposed method provides an algorithm to assign different possible doses for each subject. It helps to define the optimum dose on MTA value. It is potent enough to accumulate the doses information by capturing their variability, an overlooked area in the conventional model. A simulation study is performed to create dose values. This work is suitable for Phase-I dose without the MTD or DLT. The intention is to look for specific biomarker value by contributing effect of different doses [126]. The continual reassessment method is found suitable to work with OBD. It is detected by highest toxicity label [127]. The OBD detection technique is performed through two-stage clinical trial design [128, 129]. Further, the dose-finding design is performed with OBD by adaptive trial on molecularly targeted agents. The low-dose chemotherapy is found suitable to suppress the tumor vessel growth and controlling the damage in vascular endothelial cells [130]. The semiparametric approach proposed to detect the whole dose levels of MC by OBD [131]. In survival analysis with MCMC iteration method, the possible threshold value for OBD serves the same challenge [132].The high dose of chemotherapy with cisplatin can produce a more toxic effect [130]. The targeted MC on molecularly targeted agent works to control the vascular endothelial cells [133]. It is mentioned that new vessels generated in long-run for patients treated with the maximum tolerated dose(MTD) by angiogenesis [134]. The MTD with conventional high dose chemotherapy fails to control the growth of tumor cells by neovascularization. This drug could cause tumor neovascularity [121]. However, since the last decade, the serum creatinine is emerged as a promising surrogate marker to assess the tumor anti-angiogenesis effect [135, 136, 137, 138]. The low-dose chemotherapy is administered frequently into continuous manner to selectively suppress the vessel growth in tumor tissue and repair the damage in vascular endothelial cells (VECs) [130]. This proposed model is performed by dose-response modeling by avoiding the toxicity label in a clinical trial. The simulation study shows that the proposed model works relatively well. It is better than the parametric model. Because in MC trial, the occurrence of toxicity is limited.

```
#Model 1

model;
{
#prior distribution for beta
for(i in 1:10){beta[i]~ dnorm(0,.0001) } #Dose=X
for(i in 1:N1){for(j in 1:M1)
{Y1[i,j] ~ dnorm(mu1[i,j],tau)}
for(i in 1:N1){for(j in 1:M1)
{
mu1[i,j]<- beta[1]+beta[2] ×time1[j]+
b[i,1]+b[i,2]×time1[j]}}
for (i in 1:N5){for (j in 1:M5)mu5[i,j]<- beta[9]
+beta[10]×time4[j]+b[i,9]+b[i,10]×time5[j]}
for(i in 1:N1)b[i,1:10] ~ dmnorm(vu[],Omega[,])}
for (
i in 1:10){vu[i]<-0
Omega[1:10,1:10]{ dwish(R[,],10)
Sigma[1:10,1:10]<-inverse(Omega[,])
tau ~ dgamma(.00001,.00001)
Var<-1/tau
}
```

```
#Model 2
model;
{
beta[i] ~ dnorm(0.0, 0.001) # Dose=X
for(i in 1:N1){ for (j in 2:M1)Y1[i,j] ~ dnorm(mu1[i,j],tau) }}
for(i in 1:N1){for (j in 2:M1)
mu1[i,j]<-beta1[i]×(1-rho)+beta2[i]×(time1[j]-
rho ×time1[j-1])+rho×Y1[i,j-1]}}
for(i in 1:N1){ Y1[i,1] ~ dnorm(mu1[i,1],tau)}
for(i in 1:N1){ mu1[i,1]<-beta1+beta2 ×time1[1]}
tau ~ dgamma(.001,.001)
rho ~ dbeta(1,1)
sigma<-1/tau
}
```

Chapter 15

Concordance Analysis

Abstract

One of the parameter to promote cancer research is dependent on diagnostics technique expansion. However, every time new diagnostic technique need to test in presences of an actual diagnostic test. Several times disease measured by continuous measurement. Now concordance correlation coefficient (CCC) is one of the tools in diagnostics test statistics. It performs as a tool in agreement analysis. It supports continuous measurement. The continuous variable, i.e., tumor size measured or observed with a different diagnostic procedure, can be computed by CCC. This chapter shows the Bayesian extension of the CCC for continuous data. Now Bayes factor is illustrated by real-life data to define the best diagnostics tool. The approach illustrated in this work provides the researchers with an opportunity to find out the most appropriate model for specific data and apply CCC to fulfil the desired hypothesis.

15.1 Introduction

One of the significant proportion of oncology research is devoted to diagnostic research. The risk of misdiagnosis always stands in oncology. The diagnosis is not easy and straightforward. The complex diagnosis and differential diagnosis needs to be similar to define conclusive remark about the presence of the disease condition. Sometimes physicians make a diagnosis error. Sometimes two physicians disagree on a diagnosis among them. However, they look at the same CT scan or MRI report. It becomes confusing while compare CT scans with MRI reports. Alternatively, two physicians independently comment same or different diagnosis tets. The disease status detection is not an easy task. There is always a dilemma to define cancer staging. Due to rapid disease progression and disease complexity, it is not an easy task to detect tumor staging. Now it requires to make a conclusive remark about diagnosis test. The agreement comes while we define the diagnosis status. Since the tumor measured into size or dimension, so the tumor measurement data generated as a continuous variable. The continuous variable, i.e., tumor size measured or observed with a different diagnostic procedure can be concluded by concordance correlation, in this chapter, the concordance correlation illustrated with tumor size and tumor volume measurements. While the measured outcome defined with the binary variable, then it is presented with kappa statistics. Sometimes, the weighted kappa also useful. The 'inter-rater agreement' and 'inter-device agreement' required to quantifying the extent of agreement between two or more examiners or devices is of primary interest.Widely known as the intraclass correlation measurement is a choice [139, 140, 141]. The application of the within-subject coefficient of variation found attractive in this context [142]. Now the Inter-rater agreement is important, for example, when different raters evaluate the severity of a specific disease during a clinical trial, and the reliability of each of their subjective evaluation is to determine by measuring agreement among the raters [143].

#Concordance Correlation Coefficient

The concordance correlation coefficient ρ_c defined as

$$\rho_c = \frac{2\rho\sigma_x\sigma_y}{\sigma_x^2 + \sigma_y^2 + (\mu_x - \mu_y)^2} \qquad (15.1)$$

Now, μ_x and μ_y are the average of the two continuous variables. The term σ_x^2 and σ_y^2 are the corresponding variance. Now ρ is the correlation coefficient between the two variables.

#Concordance Correlation Coefficient for Paired Data

Similarly, it can be calculated from the paired data. If x and y variables are observed into paired manner, then the concordance correlation coefficient becomes

$$\hat{\rho}_c = \frac{2_{xy}}{2 \atop x + 2 \atop y + (\bar{x} - \bar{y})^2} \qquad (15.2)$$

The pair of observations is n.

It is always required for new diagnosis procedure to diagnose cancer more accurately. Now the challenge is to establish the accuracy of the new diagnostic tool in presences of the existing one. The concordance correlation coefficient is useful to quantify the agreement between two raters measured independently on the same subject. A new diagnostic tool promotion becomes challenging in the presence of an available tool. Now new tool needs to proof as authoritative or as equal in the presence of diagnostic tool. Now the different diagnostic tool is required to be compared to explore the agreement on measurement. Unless the new diagnostic tools are performed equal or better, we can not use in regular news. In this context, the concordance correlation coefficient becomes useful. There are different tools available on continuous data like the coefficient of variation, t-test, intra-class correlation, Pearson correlation coefficient, and least square analysis. However, these are not useful to work toward agreement analysis. There are a few limitations. The Intra-class correlation coefficient assumed that the readings between two observers are interchangeable. It is not robust enough. Now the least-squares analysis is not suitable enough for the null hypothesis in the presence of a residual error that is very large or small [144]. Similarly, the Pearson correlation is also not enough in this context. Now the concordance correlation coefficient (CCC) supports for differentiating the concordance measurement [145]. The computation of the Z-transformation is difficult. The methodological work supports that CCC provides similar to the value of the Pearson correlation coefficient if the mean and variance of the measurement of interest [144]. There is an illustration of the CCC [146]. It is based on the covariance-based index. Now the stratified CCC [147] and the generalized estimating equation is established [148]. The size of the tumor is mainly concerned in any regular or experimental cancer therapy. Determination of tumor size by diagnostic procedures is an important key indicator for any therapeutic success. Recently, several types of diagnostic procedures are available for tumor size detection like computed tomography (CT) and magnetic resonance imaging (MRI) with advanced technology. Generally, pre and post-therapy tumor size provide therapeutic results in any specific direction. It is ideal that the same diagnostic procedure should be applied to detect the tumor size before and after a therapeutic effect to reduce the diagnostic testing variation. Simultaneously, same way interpretation about tumor size needs to be performed. Broadly, two types of approaches are available for detection of tumor size, either through tumor volume or by the maximum area covered by the tumor. This chapter is about proposing the Bayesian counterpart to compute CCC for continuous data.

15.2 Computational Methodology

This data is obtained through a brain cancer diagnosis. A total of 35 patients tumor size and volume is considered in this work. Now tumor volume is measured with MRI and tumor size by CR scan. The measurements are obtained at two-time points, i.e., pre and post-surgery about tumor volume and size. In this work, the Bayesian counterpart of the concordance correlation coefficient is illustrated in this chapter. Suppose the ith reading is defined for N subjects in a study. The response vector is defined as $Y_i(i = 1, 2, ...N, i \leq I)$ for $I \times 1$ vectors that contained the I readings. Now, different methods is defined as Y_i and $Y_{i'}$ $Y_{i'}(1 \leq I, i' \leq I, I \neq i')$ respectively. The expected square different is $E[(Y_i - Y_{i'})^2]$ defined as CCC as scaled between -1 and 1.

The CCC is defined as

$$\rho_{CCC} = 1 - \frac{E[(Y_i - Y_{i'})^2]}{\sigma_i^2 + \sigma_{i'}^2 + (\mu_i - \mu_{i'})^2} = \frac{2\sigma_{ii'}}{\sigma_i^2 + \sigma_{i'}^2 + (\mu_i - \mu_i')^2} \qquad (15.3)$$

Now $E(Y_i) = \mu_i, E(Y_{i'}) = \mu_{i'}, \sigma_i^2 = var(Y_i), \sigma_{i'}^2 = var(Y_{i'})$, $\sigma_{ii'} = cov(Y_i, Y_{i'}) = \sigma_i \sigma_{i'} \rho_{ii'}$. Now the terms $S_{ii'}, s_i^2, s_{i'}^2, \bar{Y}_i$ and $\bar{Y}_{i'}$ are considered as unbiased estimates of $\sigma_{ij}, \sigma_i^2, \sigma_{i'}^2, \mu_i$ and $\mu_{i'}$ respectively. Now the expected of this estimates for k types of different methods is limited with $k = 2$ for two scanner is

$$E\left(\frac{2}{k(k-1)} \sum_{i=1}^{k-1} \sum_{i'=i+1}^{k} S_{ii'}\right) = \frac{2}{k(k-1)} \sum_{i=1}^{k-1} \sum_{i'=i+1}^{k} \sigma_{ii'} \qquad (15.4)$$

$$E\left(\frac{1}{k} \sum_{i=1}^{k} S_i^2\right) = \frac{1}{k} \sum_{i=1}^{k} \sigma_i^2 \qquad (15.5)$$

$$E\left(\frac{1}{k(k-1)} \sum_{i=1}^{k-1} \sum_{i'=i+1}^{k} (\bar{Y}_i - \bar{Y}_{i'})^2\right) = \frac{1}{k(k-1)} \sum_{i=1}^{k-1} \sum_{i'=i+1}^{k} (\mu_i - \mu_{i'})^2 + \frac{\sigma_e^2}{n} \quad (15.6)$$

Now, $\sum_{i=1}^{k-1} \sum_{i'=i+1}^{k} (\bar{Y}_i - \bar{Y}_{i'})^2$ is a biased estimator of $\sum_{i=1}^{k-1} \sum_{i'=i+1}^{k} (\mu_i - \mu_{i'})^2$.
The corresponding unbiased estimator is defined as

$$\sum_{i=1}^{k-1} \sum_{i'=i+1}^{k} (\bar{Y}_i - \bar{Y}_{i'})^2 - \frac{k(k-1)}{n} \sigma_e^2 = W - Z \qquad (15.7a)$$

$$W = \sum_{i=1}^{k-1} \sum_{i'=i+1}^{k} (\bar{Y}_i - \bar{Y}_{i'})^2 \qquad (15.7b)$$

$$Z = \frac{k(k-1)}{n} \sum_{i=1}^{k-1} \sum_{i'=i+1}^{k} (S_i^2 + S_{i'}^2 - 2S_{ii'})^2 \qquad (15.7c)$$

Finally, unbiased estimate of ρ_{CCC} is defined as $\bar{\rho}_{CCC}$

$$\bar{\rho}_{CCC} = \frac{2 \sum_{i=1}^{k-1} \sum_{i'=i+1}^{k} S_{ii'}}{P - Q} \qquad (15.8)$$

where

$$P = (k-1) \sum_{i=1}^{k} S_i^2 + \sum_{i=1}^{k-1} \sum_{i'=i+1}^{k} (\bar{Y}_i - \bar{Y}_{i'})^2 \qquad (15.9)$$

$$Q = \frac{k(k-1)}{n} \sum_{i}^{k-1} \sum_{i'=k+1}^{k} (S_i^2 + S_{i'}^2 - 2S_{ii'}) \tag{15.10}$$

Suppose i and i' represents different reading for the jth patients. The method number assigned by $k = 2$, i.e., CT Scanner and MRI Scanner. The responses are defined as Y_{ij} and $Y_{i'j}$ of the same patients $'j'$. Now the linear model for two scanners are presented as

$$Y_{ii'j} = \theta + \beta Y + \beta_i Y_i + \beta_{i'} Y_{i'} + \epsilon_{ii'j} \tag{15.11}$$

Now the continuous outcome of the measured variable is represented as $Y_{ii'j}$. The response measured for the jth individual, ith observation by kth method. The overall mean is presented as θ with mean value tumor size Y as fixed effect. The random effects are presented as Y_i and $Y_{i'}$ as random effects. The error term is presented as $\epsilon_{ii'j} \sim N(0, \tau)$. Now the term $\epsilon_{ii'j}$ is stands for precision for jth individual. The regression parameter of the fixed effect is presented with N(0.0.0001) and random effects as Gamma(0.0.0001). Further, the fixed effect variance, random effect variance and error terms are combined with equation (15.7) as

$$\sigma_{fixed}^2 = \frac{2}{k(k-1)} \sum_{i'+1}^{k-1} \sum_{i'=i+1}^{k} \sigma_{ij} \tag{15.12}$$

$$\sigma_{random}^2 = \frac{1}{k(k-1)} \sum_{i=1}^{k-1} \sum_{i'=i+1}^{k} (\mu_i - \mu_{i'})^2 \tag{15.13}$$

and

$$\sigma_{error}^2 = \frac{2}{k(k-1)} \sum_{i=1}^{k-1} \sum_{i'=i+1}^{k} \frac{1}{2}(\sigma_i^2 + \sigma_{i'}^2 - 2\sigma_{ii'})^2$$

$$= \frac{1}{k} \sum_{i=1}^{k} \sigma_i^2 - \frac{2}{k(k-1)} \sum_{i=1}^{k-1} \sum_{i=i+1}^{k} \sigma_{ii'} \tag{15.14}$$

The CCC is defined as

$$\rho_{CCC} = \frac{\sigma_{fixed}^2}{\sigma_{fixed}^2 + \sigma_{random}^2 + \sigma_{error}^2} = \frac{\sum_{i=1}^{k-1} \sum_{i'=i+1}^{k}}{(k-1) \sum_{i=1}^{k} \sum_{i'=i+1}^{k} (\mu_i - \mu_{i'})^2} \tag{15.15}$$

The term θ is constant $\sigma_{fixed}^2 = \frac{1}{\tau_f}$, $\sigma_{random}^2 = \frac{1}{\tau_r}$ and $\sigma_{error}^2 = \frac{1}{\tau_e}$. To formulate the Bayesian analysis, we assign prior on the parameters, τ_f, τ_r, τ_e as follows:

$$\theta \sim dnorm(0, 0.001) \tag{15.16}$$

$$\tau_f \sim \text{dgamma}(0.0001, 0.0001) \qquad (15.17)$$

$$\tau_r \sim \text{dnorm}(0.0001, 0.0001) \text{ and} \qquad (15.18)$$

$$\tau_e \sim \text{dgamma}(0.0001, 0.0001) \qquad (15.19)$$

15.3   Bayes Factor

Where dnorm stands for normal distribution, dgamma denotes the Gamma distribution. The parameters of the distribution considered as non-informative prior and fixed as 0 and 0.001 for normal distribution and 0.0001 and 0.0001 for Gamma distribution. The Bayesian factor is applied through JZS for Concordance Correlation in regression line [148]. The regression coefficient β is permitted to the application of JZS prior. The CCC, Intercept (θ), regression coefficients and error term ($\epsilon_{ii'j}$) are detailed in equation (15.7). Let the equation (15.7) further been separated into Model (M_1) and Model (M_0) by

$$M_1 : Y = \theta + \beta X + \epsilon_{ii'j} \qquad (15.20)$$

$$M_0 : Y = \theta + \epsilon_{ii'j} \qquad (15.21)$$

The model (M_1) states the presence of CCC and absence of it by model (M_0). Now, the Bayes Factor through JZS is defined [148, 149, 150] as,

$$BF_{10} = \frac{(n/2)^{1/2}}{\tau(1/2)} \times \int_0^\infty (1+g)^{(n-2)/2} \times [1 + (1 - r^2)g]^{-\frac{(n-1)}{2}} \qquad (15.22)$$

$$BF_{10} = \frac{p(Y(M_1)}{p(Y(M_0)} \qquad (15.23)$$

If the value of BF_{10} becomes more than 1, it states about the presences of CCC otherwise not. The statistical test can be performed with two Hypotheses: the Null Hypothesis, H_0 as given in model (M_0) and the alternative hypothesis H_1 or (M_1). The prior probability of null hypothesis is assigned as $p(M_0)$ and alternative as $p(M_1)$. Therefore, Baye's theorem is applied to the observed data to compute the posterior probability of the Hypothesis. The appearance of the posterior probability of alternative Hypothesis is computed as

$$p(M_1/Y) = \frac{p(Y|M_1)p(M_1)}{p(Y|M_1)p(M_1) + p(Y|M_0)p(M_0)} \qquad (15.24)$$

The term $P(Y|M_1)$ is the marginal likelihood of the data for alternative hypotheses. Further, the marginal likelihood is calculated as

$$p(Y|M_1) = \int_{\theta}^{\infty} p(Y|\theta, M_1)p(\theta|H_1)d\theta \tag{15.25}$$

Bayes Factor is used to compute the appearance of $P(M_1|Y)$ in comparison to $P(M_0|Y)$ [151]:

$$\frac{p(M_1|Y)}{p(M_0|Y)} = BF_{10} \times \frac{p(M_1)}{p(M_0)} \tag{15.26}$$

15.4 Results

Initially, we performed a descriptive data analysis. The classical test carried on CCC between tumor size measurements. Under the null hypothesis is assumed that the concordance correlation coefficient is zero as $\rho_{ccc} = 0$. The function named as cccUst is available in the "cccrm" package of R. Similarly, CCC is performed on tumor volume. Demographic profile of the patients provided in Table 15.1. The Bayesian posterior estimate of CCC detailed in Table 15.2 and Table 15.3. In Bayesian, the same models selected to fit the correlation coefficient to measure the association. It implies that the precision of the methods is moderate. The correlation coefficients are not very much different from calculated classical CCC detailed in Table 15.3. It can be concluded by

TABLE 15.1: Posterior estimates obtained are presented

Sex	Pre Surgery (Max,Min) (Max,Min)	Mean (SD)	Post Surgery (Max,Min)	Mean (SD)
Male	(20.83,6.08)	12.69(3.64)	(15.22,0.95)	8.33(3.42)
Female	(20.14,10.23)	13.48(3.95	(14.60,1.69)	9.38(2.81)

TABLE 15.2: Posterior Estimates of concordance correlation coefficients on tumor size

Parameter	Mean	SD	2.5%	Median	97.5%
ρ_{ccc}	0.67	0.23	0.13	0.65	0.93
σ_w^2	2.52	0.31	2.00	2.50	3.21
σ_a^2	84.22	1960.00	0.56	5.23	329.61
σ_b^2	0.01	0.024	0.00	0.00	0.06
σ_d^2	0.01	0.030	0.00	0.00	0.09
θ	3.63	2.80	-4.10	3.62	9.11

TABLE 15.3: Table 15.3:Posterior estimates of concordance correlation coefficients on tumor volume

Parameter	Mean	SD	2.5%	Median	97.5%
ρ_{ccc}	0.75	0.13	0.09	0.45	0.90
σ_w^2	11.76	1.43	9.27	11.64	14.88
σ_a^2	259.50	5528.00	1.36	13.74	992.10
σ_b^2	0.01	0.07	0.001	0.00	0.16
σ_d^2	0.01	0.03	0.00	0.00	0.07
θ	10.29	5.09	-3.84	10.63	19.95

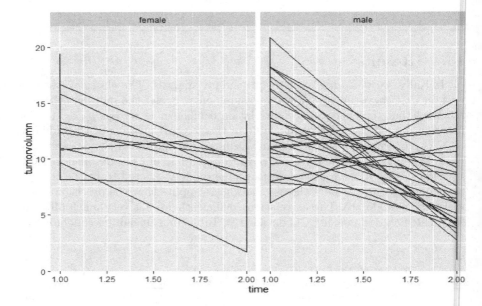

FIGURE 15.1: Tumor volume changes in both gender.

having high estimates for accuracy. The estimates obtained through Bayesian methodology is presented in Table 15.3 and Table 15.4. The same models are used to obtain the correlation coefficient to obtain the association. The result shows that the precision is moderate enough. Now the correlation coefficients are not different from calculated conventional CCC in Table 15.3 with high accuracy value. In Model 1, the posterior estimate of the concordance correlation coefficient on tumor size is obtained as 0.69. The SD is obtained as 0.23. The HPD is obtained as (0.13,0.95). Similarly, the posterior estimate on tumor volume is measured as 0.75(0.13). The HPD in a similar context is measured as (0.09,0.90). It shows that the confidence interval of the estimates is closed. Finally, the Bayes factor is measured as 9.53.

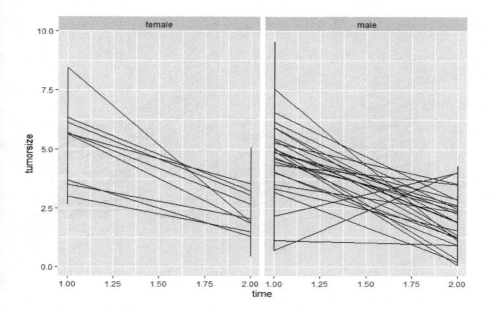

FIGURE 15.2: Tumor size changes by gender.

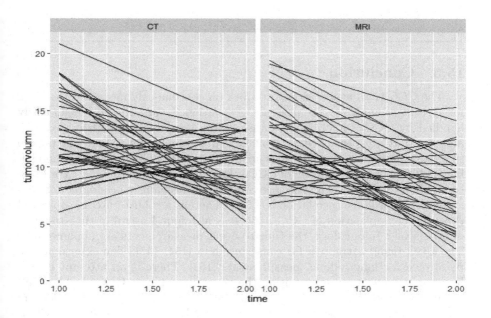

FIGURE 15.3: Tumor volume changes by both the method.

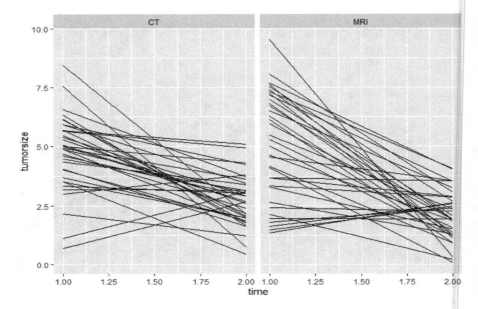

FIGURE 15.4: Tumor size changes by both the method.

15.5 Conclusion

The CCC is an available tool to work on continuously measured variables for agreement analysis. The presence of covariance, variance, and mean easily handled by CCC [146, 147]. Perhaps, it may be generated with biased estimates or in the presence of error [152]. The marginal modeling found attractive to reduce bias value [144]. There is an application of CCC by stratified modeling [153]. The wider extension of CCC is known as the generalized concordance correlation coefficient. The variance component mechanism is adopted for generalized concordance correlation by [139]. There is a robust outcome observed through the application of CCC [153]. It is also found useful in time-to-event data analysis. In oncology, the time-to-event measurements are nonignorable. The CCC found attractive for censoring data [154, 145]. The extension also performed for longitudinal measurements [151]. There is an attempt by the linear mixed effect model by using the generalized CCC (GCCC). The computational algorithm is developed to boost up the Bayesian methodology in CCC. Initially, the data fitted by GLMM and later on the Bayesian CCC is considered in this direction. It provides scope to extend it by different types of hypothesis testing. The generation of the p-value can be overlooked in this direction. The methodology on Bayesian ICC is well established [155]. As a choice, the beta bionomical model defined. It helped to generate credible intervals [156]. In this chapter, the model generated to work with MCMC. Now the technique is simple and suitable to handle continuous data. The intention is to make the Bayesian counterpart of CCC. The work is about exploring the Bayesian for CCC. Tumor volume and tumor size measurements are by CT and MRI scanner. Now the measurement obtained by MRI and CT is highly concordant. Even sometimes they replicate to each other-similarly, several diagnostic issues faced in oncology research. Now the Bayesian is functional for strong evidence on test statistics about the variables. Now the Bayes factor is used for computing the CCC. This approach promotes the different dimension of the hypothesis testing.

Chapter 16

High-Dimensional Data Analysis

Abstract

Currently, the proliferation of knowledge of cancer promotes cancer management by gene therapy. High-dimensional data measure genomic information of cancer patients. Motivated by these essential applications in cancer research, there has been a dramatic growth in the development of statistical methodology in the analysis of high-dimensional data, mainly related to regression model selection, estimation and prediction. The high-dimensional data is useful to explore the cancer progression, especially for disease management. However, the analyst faces difficulties to deal with high-dimensional data where the feature dimension p grows exponentially. This chapter is dedicated to shows the Bayesian approach in high-dimensional data. Variable selection in high-dimensional data is one of the challenges. Bayesian variable selection strategy is presented in this work. Different R packages for variable selection steps are illustrated. This chapter will help to consider Bayesian in high-dimensional variable selection.

16.1 Introduction

The base sequence procedure is now well developed. A large amount of genetic data is available publically. This large amount of data challenged us for the development of analytical tools for analyzing such accumulated data. It is essential to analyze such extensive genetic data by advanced computational methodology coupled with statistical techniques for processing genetic data. Similarly, microarray also provides gene expression information. Commonly, ten of thousands of variables obtained by a single experiment. Dataset with this large number of variables are known as high-dimensional data. Earlier, this used to measure gene expression in serum or tissue. Currently, it used for DNA methylation expression. Tremendous progress in a microarray experiment observed. Similar, growth in the statistical analysis method followed. Primarily, the gene effect classification is the main challenge in high-dimensional data analysis. Filter out a few variables from ten of thousands of variables is the task of the gene classification. The conventional approach for statistical methodology is known as an unsupervised approach. But currently, the direction shifted from unsupervised to supervised approach. The supervised approach help to define the characteristics (Y) to gene expression data (X).

The objective of high-dimensional data analysis is to make clusters between the observations. The preparation of clustering is useful to merge the representation into a similar group of individuals. It is required to take a similar type of treatment decision for the same cluster. There are different types of clustering methods, and we will explore through R.However, the statistical model is useful to predict an individual for specific clustering. Mainly, it is known as a predictive model for survival data. The method is useful, like penalized partial log-likelihood (PLL) for the estimation of the regression coefficients. The widely adopted method is lasso [157, 158]. The lasso defines the L1 penalty function. The amount of variations of the penalization is presented as SCAD [159, 160]. Other methods like the elastic net [161] and Dantzig selector[162]. The dimension reduction is also useful and can define by $p \geq n$. Methods like tree-based methods, as random survival forests [163] now well explored. The conventional approach stands with a Cox proportional hazards model. It works with time-to-event data. The procedure is to use the predictive PLL and after that, the cross-validation. It helps to variable selections from a ten of thousand of variable [164]. As an alternative to the PLL, the prediction error curve works well [165]. It helps by identifying the probabilities of survival from a risk prediction model. The prediction of the error curve is obtained by the expected squared difference of the risk prediction with actual event status by Brier score at a given time point. In a Cox regression model, there is a possibility to obtain unstable estimated regression coefficients. But stability can be achieved by maximizing the penalized partial log-likelihood. A penalty function of the regression coefficients subtracted from the partial log-likelihood. It helps to choose the optimal weight of the penalty function through maximizing the predictive value of the model [165].

16.2   Heatmap with R

```
#R Code to Prepare Heatmap

df<-read.csv("import the data",header=TRUE)
geneExpmatrix <- as.matrix(df[2:25])
head(geneExpmatrix)
heatmap.2(geneExpmatrix)
```

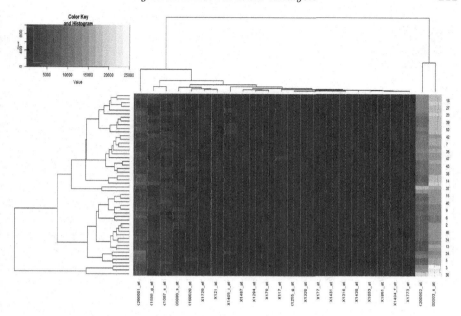

FIGURE 16.1: Heatmap in high-dimensional data.

```
#R Code for Stepwise Approach Tree Cutting

hr<-hclust(as.dist(1-cor(t(geneExpmatrix),method="pearson")),
method="complete")
hc<-hclust(as.dist(1-cor(geneExpmatrix,method="spearman")),
method="complete")
mycl<-cutree(hr, h=max(hr$height)/1.5)
mycolhc<-rainbow(length(unique(mycl)),start=0.1,end=0.9)
mycolhc<-mycolhc[as.vector(mycl)]
mycol<-colorpanel(40,"darkblue","yellow","white")
heatmap.2(geneExpmatrix,Rowv=as.dendrogram(hr),
Colv=as.dendrogram(hc),col=mycol,scale="row",density.info=
"none",trace="none"RowSideColors=mycolhc)
```

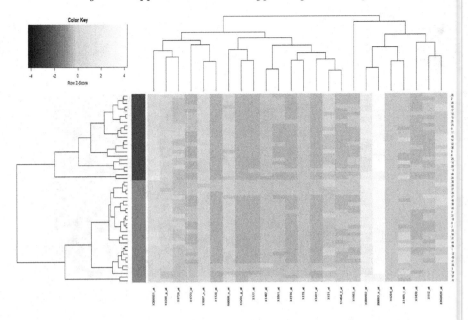

FIGURE 16.2: Stepwise approach tree cutting with R.

16.3   Principal Component Analysis with R

In this procedure, the first principal component axis and thereafter second components are obtained by looking at the eigenvalue between different variables. In this example, we illustrate the analysis of the principal component analysis (PCA) as a data reduction technique to simplify reducing the multidimensional data sets of 2 or 3 dimensions by plotting the purposes through variance analysis. Initially, the first principal component axis and thereafter second components are obtained by exploring the eigenvalue between different variables. The same

```
#R Code for Principal Component Analysis

library("gplots")
df<-read.csv("import the data from hard drive.csv", header=TRUE)
geneExpmatrix <- as.matrix(df[2:25])
pca <- prcomp(geneExpmatrix, scale=T)
summary(pca)
plot(pca$x, pch=20, col="blue", type="n")
text(pca$x, rownames(pca$x), cex=0.8)
```

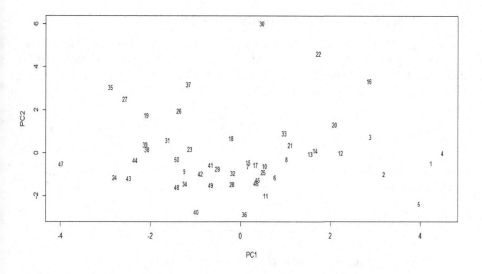

FIGURE 16.3: Principle component analysis with R.

16.4   Penalized Partial Log-Likelihood (PLL)

The penalized partial log-likelihood (PLL) is an extension of the Cox proportional hazards model

$$\lambda(t|Z_j) = \lambda_0(t)\exp(Z_i'\beta) \tag{16.1}$$

for the hazard $\lambda(t|Z_i)$, i.e., the instantaneous risk of having an event at time t, given the covariate information in Z_i, for individual i. The $\lambda_0(t)$ is used for baseline hazard function. Suppose the parameter vector $beta = (\beta_1, ..., \beta_p)'$ is defined by maximizing the PLL with

$$J(\beta) = \sum_{i=1}^{n} \delta_i(z_i'\beta - \log(\sum_{j=1}^{n} J(t_j \geq t_i)\exp(z_j'\beta))) \tag{16.2}$$

It is used as indicator function J. Now, $J(A) = 1$, if A is true, and $J(A) = 0$ otherwise. Further, the direct maximization of the PLL is not permissible if the number of covariates p is larger than the number of observations n. There are several approaches that are developed by random survival forests [166]. The PLL is useful to consider the performance of new data after model complexity is settled.

16.5   Estimating the Predictive PLL

The prediction performance of PLL is obtained by leave-one-out cross-validation procedure [166]. The 10-fold cross-validation is prescribed [167]. Now the B cross-validation splots the PLL into a new dataset by predictive PLL and it is estimated as

$$J_{\text{pred}}(\hat{\beta}) = \sum_{b=1}^{B} \sum_{i:x_i \in x_b} \delta_i (z_i' \hat{\beta}_b - \log(\sum_{j:x_j \in x_b} J(t_j \geq t_i) \exp(z_j' \hat{\beta}_{b-}))) \quad (16.3)$$

Now the estimated vector of coefficients are fitted by $\hat{\beta}_{b-}$ after leaving the bth part of the data out. Now, x_b is the bth part of the data with $b = 1, ..., B$.

16.6   Integrated Prediction Error Curve (IPEC)

The risk prediction model is defined from the fitted Cox proportional hazard model up to time t, given the covariate information z_i is

$$\hat{r}(t|z_i) = \exp(-\hat{\Delta}_0(t) \exp(z_i' \hat{\beta})) \quad (16.4)$$

The Breslow estimator $\hat{\Delta}_0$ is used to define the baseline hazard

$$\Delta_0(t) = \int_0^t \lambda_0(s) ds \quad (16.5)$$

The time-dependent measure of the prediction error can be defined by Brier score as

$$BS(t, \hat{r}) = E(Y(t) - \hat{r}(t|z_i))^2 \quad (16.6)$$

The true event status is defined as $Y(t) = J(T > t)$ at time t. The predicted event status is formulated as $\hat{r}(t|z_i)$ at that time.

16.7   Ridge Estimators in Cox Regression

Suppose the dimension is defined as $p \geq\geq n$. It is possible to handle with the Cox model. The sample size is n. Further, the follow-up time is defined as $t_1, t_2, ...t_n$. The death event indicator is defined as $d_1, ...d_n$. If $d_i = 1$ then event occured otherwise not. Now for the individual's the dimension is p as an explanatory variable. It can be presented as p-vectors $X_1; ::::; X_n$, which are the rows of the design matrix X. The proportional hazards (PH) model can be defined as

$$h(t|X_i) = h_0(t)\exp(X_i^T \beta) \tag{16.7}$$

The vector of the regression coefficients R can be defined by maximizing the partial log-likelihood as

$$pl(\beta) = \sum_{i=1}^{n} d_i (X_i^T \beta) - \ln(\sum_{t_j \geq t_i} \exp(X_j^T \beta)) \tag{16.8}$$

Suppose the baseline hazard function is defined as $h_0(t)$. Suppose the event point is defined as t_i with $d_i = 1$. Further, the Breslow estimator can be formulated as

$$\hat{h}_0(t_i) = 1/ \sum_{t_j \geq t_j} \exp(X_j^T \hat{\beta}) \tag{16.9}$$

Further, the total likelihood as combination of Breslow estimator and the partial likelihood is defined as

$$l(\beta, h_0) = \sum_{i=1}^{n} [-\exp(X_i^T \beta) H_0(t_i) + d_i((h_0(t_i)) + X_i^T \beta)] \tag{16.10}$$

with

$$H_0(t) = \sum_{s \leq t} h_0(S) \tag{16.11}$$

This model with $p >> n$ helps to fit large coefficients as $|\hat{\beta}_k| \to \infty$. It is perfect to fit as $pl(\hat{\beta}) = 0$), to degenerate baseline hazard and filter out no useful prediction model. This problem can be handled by principle component analysis by using the dimension reduction method.

$$l_{pen}(\beta, h_0) = l(\beta, h_0) - 0.5\lambda\beta^T \beta(\lambda \geq 0) \tag{16.12}$$

This is equivalent to putting the same penalty on the partial log-likelihood

$$pl_{pen}(\beta) = pl(\beta) - 0.5\lambda\beta^T \beta \tag{16.13}$$

Ridge regression works as a trad-off between bias and variance. It shows that there is an advantage in terms of the mean squared error (MSE) because $(\delta\text{MSE}/\delta\lambda) < 0$ at $\lambda = 0$.

16.8 High-Dimensional Data Analysis Using R

In this section, we will illustrate about Bayesian Variable Selection in High-Dimensional Settings by Nonlocal Priors. The BVSNLP package available in

R will be used to make the illustration. The Bayesian approach is available in this package for variable selection from high-dimensional data. It helps through the exploits mixture of point masses at zero and nonlocal priors to improve the performance of variable selection and coefficient estimation. The and product-moment (pMOM)and product inverse moment (piMOM) nonlocal priors are available for analysis. However, the binary response and survival duration is used in this package. It is possible to perform Bayesian variable selection method by Highest Posterior Probability Model (HPPM), Median Probability Model (MPM) and posterior inclusion probability for each of the covariates in the model. The data preparation steps are provided in the "Parameters Initialization" section. Different covariates are survival duration, and death status is given in this section. The cox − bvs function is useful to deliver the model. Finally, the number of model performed can be observed by length(coxout$hash$_{key}$) function. Delivraible selected model is obtained by which (coxout$max-model > 0). The idea about unnormalized probability of the selected model is obtained by (coxout$max-model > 0).

```
#Parameters Initialization

library("BVSNLP")
n <- 100
p <- 40
set.seed(123)
Sigma <- diag(p)
full <- matrix(c(rep(0.5, p*p)), ncol=p)
Sigma <- full + 0.5* Sigma
cholS <- chol(Sigma)
Beta <- c(-1.8, 1.2, -1.7, 1.4, -1.4, 1.3)
X = matrix(rnorm(n×p), ncol=p)
X = X X <- scale(X)
beta <- numeric(p)
beta[c(1:length(Beta))] <- Beta
XB <- X
surtimes < −rexp(n,exp(XB))
censtimes <- rexp(n,0.2)
times <- pmin(surtimes,censtimes)
status <- as.numeric(surtimes <= censtimes)
exmat <- cbind(times,status,X)
L <- 10; J <- 10
d <- 2 * ceiling(log(p))
temps <- seq(3, 1, length.out = L)
tau <- 0.5; r <- 1; a <- 6; b <- p-a
nlptype <- 0
cur_cols <- c(1,2,3)
nf <- 0
```

```
# Runthe Function
```

```
coxout <- cox_bvs(exmat,cur_cols,nf,tau,r,nlptype,
                  a,b,d,L,J,temps)
summary(coxout)
```

```
#Output with Function
```

```
              Length Class  Mode
max_model       40    -none- numeric
hash_key       156    -none- numeric
max_prob         1    -none- numeric
all_probs      156    -none- numeric
vis_covs_list  156    -none- list
```

```
#The Number of Visited Model for This Specific Run
```

```
length(coxouthash_key)
```

```
#Specify Model Length
```

```
length(coxout$hash_key)
[1] 156
```

```
#The Selected Model
```

```
which(coxoutmax_model}>0)
```

```
#Number of Model Selected
```

```
which(coxout$max_model>0)
[1] 1 2 3 4 5 6
```

```
#The Unnormalized Probability of the Selected Model
```

```
coxoutmax_prob
[1] -247.6858
```

#Bayesian Variable Selection in High-Dimensional Settings Using

```
library("BVSNLP")
n <- 200
p <- 40
set.seed(123)
Sigma <- diag(p)
full <- matrix(c(rep(0.5, p×p)), ncol=p)
Sigma <- full + 0.5×Sigma
cholS <- chol(Sigma)
Beta <- c(-1.7,1.8,2.5)
X <- matrix(rnorm(n×p), ncol=p)
X <- X×cholS
colnames(X) <- c(paste("gene_",c(1:p),sep=" "))
beta <- numeric(p)
beta[c(1:length(Beta))]<-Beta
Xout <- PreProcess(X)
X <- Xout$X
XB <- X×beta
probs <- as.vector(exp(XB)/(1+exp(XB)))
y <- rbinom(n,1,probs)
X <- as.data.frame(X)
train_idx <- sample(1:n,0.×n)
test_idx <- setdiff(1:n,train_idx)
X_train <- X[train_idx,]
y_train <- y[train_idx]
bout <- bvs(X_train, y_train, prep=FALSE,
family="logistic",
mod_prior ="beta",niter=50)
BMAout<-predBMA(bout,X,y,prep=FALSE,logT=FALSE,
train_idx=train_idx,test_idx=test_idx,
family="logistic")
```

#AUC for the Prediction

```
BMAout$auc
0.6953545
```

```
#BMA Prediction

$auc
[1] 0.6953545

$roc_curve
              TPR          FPR
 [1,] 1.00000000 1.00000000
 [2,] 0.89248140 0.98816334
 [3,] 0.83054193 0.97708525
 [4,] 0.83054193 0.94737135
 [5,] 0.77365963 0.94283795
 [6,] 0.73734265 0.94283795
 [7,] 0.70102566 0.93996391
 [8,] 0.66470867 0.93708988
 [9,] 0.62839169 0.93708988
[10,] 0.60986843 0.88243937
[11,] 0.54350027 0.88019476
[12,] 0.54075684 0.85048086
[13,] 0.54075684 0.82076696
[14,] 0.50443986 0.82076696
[15,] 0.49018789 0.76967992
[16,] 0.47424697 0.72165646
[17,] 0.47424697 0.69194256
[18,] 0.46870614 0.66222866
[19,] 0.43238916 0.66222866
[20,] 0.39607217 0.66222866
[21,] 0.35975518 0.66222866
[22,] 0.35426833 0.62798136
[23,] 0.31795135 0.62798136
[24,] 0.30924020 0.56879746
[25,] 0.27292322 0.56167016
[26,] 0.27292322 0.53195626
[27,] 0.26252634 0.48879049
[28,] 0.25072939 0.44575389
[29,] 0.20422736 0.43512925
[30,] 0.20422736 0.39891747
[31,] 0.20422736 0.36920357
[32,] 0.20422736 0.32873852
[33,] 0.15120017 0.31770459
[34,] 0.13694820 0.27798936
[35,] 0.12290807 0.22769629
[36,] 0.08307837 0.21862949
[37,] 0.03847714 0.21070557
[38,] 0.02744947 0.15743430
[39,] 0.02169358 0.12772040
[40,] 0.01818087 0.09163778
[41,] 0.01298243 0.04376265
[42,] 0.00000000 0.00000000
```

```
#Plotting ROC Curve

roc <- BMAout$roc_curve
plot(roc)
```

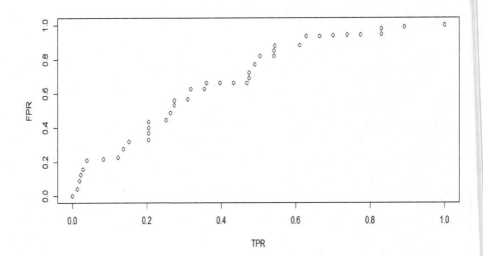

FIGURE 16.4: True positive rate and false positive rate relation.

```
#Install Packages with R for High-Dimensional Survival Analysis

install.packages("glmnet")
install.packages("Matrix")
install.packages("tidyverse")
install.packages("broom")
install.packages("survival")
```

```
#Load Packages

library("glmnet")
library("Matrix")
library("tidyverse")
library("broom")
library("survival")
```

```
#Generate toy Survival Data
```

```
time<-rnorm(100,54,10) #Survival Duration data
status<-rbinom(100,1,.5)} # Survival status data
x.1<-rnorm(100,4,.2) }  # x.1 to x.10 are ten variables
x.2<-rnorm(100,5,.18)
x.3<-rnorm(100,6,.29)
x.4<-rnorm(100,7,.26)
x.5<-rnorm(100,8,.22)
x.6<-rnorm(100,9,.29)
x.7<-rnorm(100,10,.26)
x.8<-rnorm(100,11,.12)
x.9<-rnorm(100,12,.22)
x.10<-rnorm(100,13,.3))
```

```
Reformed the x.1 to x.10 Variables into Matrix
```

```
fdata<-data.frame(x.1,x.2,x.3,x.4,x.5,x.6,x.7,x.8,x.9,x.10)
x <- fdata %>% select(x.1,x.2,x.3,x.4,x.5,x.6,x.7,x.8,x.9
,x.10)
 %>% data.matrix()
```

```
#Output1
```

```
cv.fit2   =cv.glmnet(x,Surv(time,status),alpha  =  1,  family  =
"cox",maxit =1000) plot(cv.fit2)
```

```
#Output2
```

```
log(cv.fit2$lambda.min)
-2.229185
cv.fit2$lambda.min
0.1076161
```

```
#Output3
```

```
est.coef = coef(cv.fit2, s = cv.fit2$lambda.min)
active.k = which(est.coef != 0)
active.k
integer(0)
```

```
#Output4
```

```
active.k.vals = est.coef[active.k]
active.k.vals
numeric(0)
```

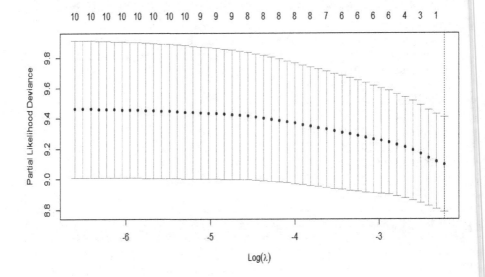

FIGURE 16.5: Partial likelihood estimates.

16.9 Different Packages with R

16.9.1 BAMA

```
#R Code for Shrinkage Estimator on High-Dimensional Datadd

install.packages("bama")
library(bama) # call the library bma#
Y <- bama.data$y # generate continous variable of size 1000#
A <- bama.data$ a # generate continous variable of size 1000#
M <- as.matrix(bama.data[, paste0("m", 1:100)],
nrow(bama.data))
#Create the Matrix of having M#
C1 <- matrix(1, 1000, 1) #Create one covariate of C1#
C2 <- matrix(1, 1000, 1)#Create one covariate of C2#
beta.m <- rep(0, 100)
alpha.a <- rep(0, 100)
set.seed(12345)
#bama function is used filter influencing variable in the regression#
out<-bama(Y,A,M,C1,C2,beta.m,alpha.a,burnin=1000,
ndraws = 100)
summary <- summary(out)
head(summary)
```

16.9.2   countgmifs

This package is useful to fit negative binomial nd Poisson regression by stagewise manner. It is illustrated in the following text:

```
#R Code on Countgmifsp

install.packages("countgmifs")
library("countgmifs")
set.seed(10)
n <- 50 # Sample size of the data
p <- 500 #Covariates required for the data
intercept<- .5
#generate parameter for 500 covariates#
beta<- c(log(1.5), log(1.5),
-log(1.5), -log(1.5),
-log(1.5), rep(0,495))
alpha<- 0.5 # Intercept
x<- matrix(rnorm(n×p,0,1), nrow=n, ncol=p,
byrow=TRUE) #Covariate values
colnames(x)<- paste("Var",1:p, sep=" ")
mu<- exp(intercept + crossprod(t(x),beta))
y<- rnbinom(n=n, size=1/alpha ,mu=mu) # Discrete response
data<- data.frame(y,x)
nb<-countgmifs(y  1 , data=data, offset=NULL,
x=x, epsilon=0.01, tol=0.001,
scale=TRUE, verbose=FALSE)
coef.AIC<-coef(nb, model.select="AIC")
coef.AIC[coef.AIC!=0]
predict(nb, model.select="AIC")
plot(predict(nb, model.select="AIC"), y)
plot(nb)
```

16.9.3   fastcox

This R package is used for Lasso and Elastic-Net Penalized Cox's Regression in High Dimensions Models by the Cocktail Algorithm. In this package, the majorization-minimization principle is applied of the elastic net penalized Cox's proportional hazard model. It is illustrated on the following page.

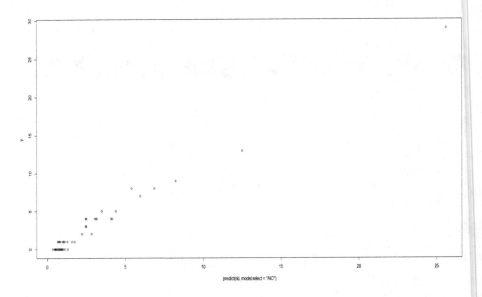

FIGURE 16.6: Model selection by AIC.

```
#R Code on Fastcox

install.packages("fastcox")
library("fastcox")
data(FHT)
m1<-cocktail(x=FHT$x,y=FHT$y,d=FHT$status,alpha=0.5)
predict(m1,type="nonzero")
plot(m1)
plot(m1,xvar="lambda",label=TRUE)
plot(m1,color=TRUE)
```

16.9.4   HighDimOut

The HighDimOut package is useful for Outlier Detection Algorithms in High-Dimensional Data. It is helpful for outlier detection by unification scheme. One example of running this package is detailed.

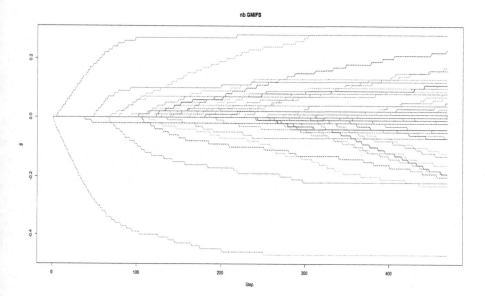

FIGURE 16.7: plot predicted values.

```
#R Code to Run HighDimOut

library("HighDimOut")
library("ggplot2")
res.ABOD <- Func.ABOD(data=TestData[,1:2], basic=FALSE,
perc=0.2)
data.temp <- TestData[,1:2]
data.temp$Ind <- NA
data.temp[order(res.ABOD,
decreasing = FALSE)[1:10],"Ind"]
<- "Outlier"
data.temp[is.na(data.temp$Ind),"Ind"] <- "Inlier"
data.temp$Ind <- factor(data.temp$Ind)
ggplot(data = data.temp) + geom_point(aes(x = x, y = y,
color=Ind, shape=Ind))
```

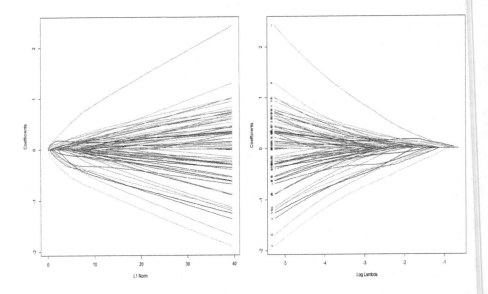

FIGURE 16.8: prediction of L1 norm and log lambda.

16.10　Discussion

Data science is an emerging field in oncology. Due to the availability of huge gene data, it can not be avoided. Always analyst faces difficulties to deal with high-dimensional data where the feature dimension p grows exponentially. The sample size is fixed at n, but $\log(p) = 0(n^{\alpha})$ for some $\alpha \in (0, 1/2)$. Currently, modern technology, like microarray analysis and next-generation sequencing data is available to generate genomics data. Large amounts of data containing more than thousands of variables are available. It is common to collect gene expressions from $p > 20{,}000$ genomics studies. These genomics data are having a large sample size and a limited size p parameter. The large size gene data analysis is a challenge. Consideration of not relevant features in the statistical literature indeed may provide undesirable computing challenges. The challenges are handled by variable screening and selection techniques. Among all methodological development, the penalized approach is favored by researchers with K-fold cross-validation.

Bibliography

[1] Shashi Kant Mishra and Bhagwat Ram. *Introduction to Unconstrained Optimization with R*. Springer Nature, 2019.

[2] John M Lachin and Mary A Foulkes. Evaluation of sample size and power for analyses of survival with allowance for nonuniform patient entry, losses to follow-up, noncompliance, and stratification. *Biometrics*, pages 507–519, 1986.

[3] Evangelos Briasoulis, Periklis Pappas, Christian Puozzo, Christos Tolis, George Fountzilas, Urania Dafni, Marios Marselos, and Nicholas Pavlidis. Dose-ranging study of metronomic oral vinorelbine in patients with advanced refractory cancer. *Clinical cancer research*, 15(20):6454–6461, 2009.

[4] Vincent T DeVita and Edward Chu. A history of cancer chemotherapy. *Cancer research*, 68(21):8643–8653, 2008.

[5] Howard E Skipper, Frank M Schabel Jr, L Bruce Mellett, John A Montgomery, Lee J Wilkoff, Harris H Lloyd, and R Wallace Brockman. Implications of biochemical, cytokinetic, pharmacologic, and toxicologic relationships in the design of optimal therapeutic schedules. *Cancer chemother Rep*, 54(6):431–450, 1970.

[6] Pan Pantziarka, Lisa Hutchinson, Nicolas André, Sébastien Benzekry, Francesco Bertolini, Atanu Bhattacharjee, Shubhada Chiplunkar, Dan G Duda, Vikram Gota, Sudeep Gupta, et al. Next generation metronomic chemotherapy-report from the fifth biennial international metronomic and anti-angiogenic therapy meeting, 6–8 may 2016, mumbai. *ecancermedicalscience*, 10, 2016.

[7] Fred Ederer. The relative survival rate: a statistical methodology. *NCI monograph*, 6:101–121, 1961.

[8] Francesca De Felice, Daniela Musio, and Vincenzo Tombolini. Head and neck cancer: metronomic chemotherapy. *BMC cancer*, 15(1):677, 2015.

[9] Peter Schmid, Walter Schippinger, Thorsten Nitsch, Gerdt Huebner, Volker Heilmann, Wolfgang Schultze, Hubert Hausmaninger, Manfred Wischnewsky, and Kurt Possinger. Up-front tandem high-dose

chemotherapy compared with standard chemotherapy with doxorubicin and paclitaxel in metastatic breast cancer: results of a randomized trial. *Journal of clinical oncology*, 23(3):432–440, 2005.

[10] Douglas Hanahan, Gabriele Bergers, and Emily Bergsland. Less is more, regularly: metronomic dosing of cytotoxic drugs can target tumor angiogenesis in mice. *The Journal of clinical investigation*, 105(8):1045–1047, 2000.

[11] Leonard B Saltz. Progress in cancer care: the hope, the hype, and the gap between reality and perception. *Journal of clinical oncology*, 26(31):5020–5021, 2008.

[12] YA Luqmani. Mechanisms of drug resistance in cancer chemotherapy. *Medical principles and practice*, 14(Suppl. 1):35–48, 2005.

[13] RS Kerbel, G Klement, KI Pritchard, and B Kamen. Continuous low-dose anti-angiogenic/metronomic chemotherapy: from the research laboratory into the oncologyclinic, 2002.

[14] Ross L Prentice, John D Kalbfleisch, Arthur V Peterson Jr, Nancy Flournoy, Vernon T Farewell, and Norman E Breslow. The analysis of failure times in the presence of competing risks. *Biometrics*, pages 541–554, 1978.

[15] John D Kalbfleisch and Ross L Prentice. *The statistical analysis of failure time data*, volume 360. John Wiley & Sons, 2011.

[16] Rebecca Gelman, Richard Gelber, I Craig Henderson, C Norman Coleman, and Jay R Harris. Improved methodology for analyzing local and distant recurrence. *Journal of clinical oncology*, 8(3):548–555, 1990.

[17] Richard J Caplan, Thomas F Pajak, and James D Cox. Analysis of the probability and risk of cause-specific failure. *International journal of radiation oncology* biology* physics*, 29(5):1183–1186, 1994.

[18] Ted A Gooley, Wendy Leisenring, John Crowley, and Barry E Storer. Estimation of failure probabilities in the presence of competing risks: new representations of old estimators. *Statistics in medicine*, 18(6):695–706, 1999.

[19] Martin G Larson and Gregg E Dinse. A mixture model for the regression analysis of competing risks data. *Journal of the royal statistical society: series C (Applied Statistics)*, 34(3):201–211, 1985.

[20] Jason P Fine and Robert J Gray. A proportional hazards model for the subdistribution of a competing risk. *Journal of the american statistical association*, 94(446):496–509, 1999.

[21] Per Kragh Andersen, John P Klein, and Susanne Rosthøj. Generalised linear models for correlated pseudo-observations, with applications to multi-state models. *Biometrika*, 90(1):15–27, 2003.

[22] Bernhard Haller, Georg Schmidt, and Kurt Ulm. Applying competing risks regression models: an overview. *Lifetime data analysis*, 19(1):33–58, 2013.

[23] Leo Breiman. Random forests. *Machine learning*, 45(1):5–32, 2001.

[24] Hemant Ishwaran, Thomas A Gerds, Udaya B Kogalur, Richard D Moore, Stephen J Gange, and Bryan M Lau. Random survival forests for competing risks. *Biostatistics*, 15(4):757–773, 2014.

[25] G Schwarz. Estimating the dimension of a model. annals of statistics, 6 (2), 461–464, 1978.

[26] H Akaike. hon entropy maximization principle. iin pr krishnarah (ed.), applications of statistics. *Amsterdam: NorthjHolland*, 1977.

[27] John P Klein and Melvin L Moeschberger. *Survival analysis: techniques for censored and truncated data.* Springer Science & Business Media, 2006.

[28] Luc Duchateau and Paul Janssen. *The frailty model.* Springer science & business media, 2007.

[29] Philip Hougaard. Shared frailty models. In *Analysis of multivariate survival data*, pages 215–262. Springer, 2000.

[30] José Cortiñas Abrahantes, Catherine Legrand, Tomasz Burzykowski, Paul Janssen, Vincent Ducrocq, and Luc Duchateau. Comparison of different estimation procedures for proportional hazards model with random effects. *Computational statistics & data analysis*, 51(8):3913–3930, 2007.

[31] Virginie Rondeau, Yassin Mazroui, and Juan R Gonzalez. frailtypack: an R package for the analysis of correlated survival data with frailty models using penalized likelihood estimation or parametrical estimation. *Journal of statistical software*, 47(4):1–28, 2012.

[32] Terry Therneau. coxme: mixed effects cox models. R package version 2.2-3. *Vienna, Austria: R Foundation for Statistical Computing*, 2012.

[33] Il Do Ha, Maengseok Noh, and Youngjo Lee. frailtyhl: A package for fitting frailty models with h-likelihood. *The R Journal*, 4(2):28–36, 2012.

[34] Marco Munda, Federico Rotolo, Catherine Legrand, et al. Parfm: parametric frailty models in uppercaseR. *Journal of statistical software*, 51(11):1–20, 2012.

[35] Andreas Wienke. *Frailty models in survival analysis.* CRC press, 2010.

[36] Ronald T Cotton, Hop S Tran Cao, Abbas A Rana, Yvonne H Sada, David A Axelrod, John A Goss, Mark A Wilson, Steven A Curley, and Nader N Massarweh. Impact of the treating hospital on care outcomes for hepatocellular carcinoma. *Hepatology*, 68(5):1879–1889, 2018.

[37] Evan M Graboyes, Mark A Ellis, Hong Li, John M Kaczmar, Anand K Sharma, Eric J Lentsch, Terry A Day, and Chanita Hughes Halbert. Racial and ethnic disparities in travel for head and neck cancer treatment and the impact of travel distance on survival. *Cancer*, 124(15):3181–3191, 2018.

[38] Yuhui Chen, Timothy Hanson, and Jiajia Zhang. Accelerated hazards model based on parametric families generalized with bernstein polynomials. *Biometrics*, 70(1):192–201, 2014.

[39] Haiming Zhou and Timothy Hanson. A unified framework for fitting bayesian semiparametric models to arbitrarily censored survival data, including spatially referenced data. *Journal of the american statistical association*, 113(522):571–581, 2018.

[40] T Hakulinen and L Tenkanen. Regression analysis of relative survival rates. *Journal of the royal statistical society: series C (applied statistics)*, 36(3):309–317, 1987.

[41] Arun Pokhrel and Timo Hakulinen. Age-standardisation of relative survival ratios of cancer patients in a comparison between countries, genders and time periods. *European journal of cancer*, 45(4):642–647, 2009.

[42] PC Lambert, PW Dickman, CP Nelson, and P Royston. Estimating the crude probability of death due to cancer and other causes using relative survival models. *Statistics in medicine*, 29(7-8):885–895, 2010.

[43] Klemen Pavlič and Maja Pohar Perme. On comparison of net survival curves. *BMC medical research methodology*, 17(1):79, 2017.

[44] Klemen Pavlič and Maja Pohar Perme. Using pseudo-observations for estimation in relative survival. *Biostatistics*, 20(3):384–399, 2019.

[45] Maja Pohar Perme, Janez Stare, and Jacques Estève. On estimation in relative survival. *Biometrics*, 68(1):113–120, 2012.

[46] Paola Rebora, Stefania Galimberti, and Maria Grazia Valsecchi. Using multiple timescale models for the evaluation of a time-dependent treatment. *Statistics in medicine*, 34(28):3648–3660, 2015.

[47] Margaret Sullivan Pepe and Motomi Mori. Kaplan-meier, marginal or conditional probability curves in summarizing competing risks failure time data? *Statistics in medicine*, 12(8):737–751, 1993.

[48] Yi-Ching Yao. Maximum likelihood estimation in hazard rate models with a change-point. *Communications in statistics-theory and methods*, 15(8):2455–2466, 1986.

[49] JD Buckley. Additive and multiplicative models for relative survival rates. *Biometrics*, pages 51–62, 1984.

[50] Janez Stare, Robin Henderson, and Maja Pohar. An individual measure of relative survival. *Journal of the royal statistical society: series C (applied statistics)*, 54(1):115–126, 2005.

[51] Douglas Bates, Martin Maechler, Ben Bolker, Steven Walker, Rune Haubo Bojesen Christensen, Henrik Singmann, Bin Dai, Gabor Grothendieck, Peter Green, and Maintainer Ben Bolker. Package lme4. *Convergence*, 12(1):2, 2015.

[52] David Clayton. Some approaches to the analysis of recurrent event data. *Statistical methods in medical research*, 3(3):244–262, 1994.

[53] Hemant Ishwaran and Lancelot F James. Computational methods for multiplicative intensity models using weighted gamma processes: proportional hazards, marked point processes, and panel count data. *Journal of the american statistical association*, 99(465):175–190, 2004.

[54] Alan E Gelfand and Adrian FM Smith. Sampling-based approaches to calculating marginal densities. *Journal of the american statistical association*, 85(410):398–409, 1990.

[55] Bradley P Carlin, Alan E Gelfand, and Adrian FM Smith. Hierarchical bayesian analysis of changepoint problems. *Journal of the royal statistical society: series C (applied statistics)*, 41(2):389–405, 1992.

[56] Nicholas Lange, Bradley P Carlin, and Alan E Gelfand. Hierarchical bayes models for the progression of hiv infection using longitudinal cd4 t-cell numbers. *Journal of the american statistical association*, 87(419):615–626, 1992.

[57] Siddhartha Chib and Bradley P Carlin. On mcmc sampling in hierarchical longitudinal models. *Statistics and computing*, 9(1):17–26, 1999.

[58] Vanita Noronha, Vijay M Patil, Amit Joshi, Atanu Bhattacharjee, Davinder Paul, Sachin Dhumal, Shashikant Juvekar, Supreeta Arya, and Kumar Prabhash. A tertiary care experience with paclitaxel and cetuximab as palliative chemotherapy in platinum sensitive and nonsensitive in head and neck cancers. *South asian journal of cancer*, 6(1):11, 2017.

[59] Shanshan Li. Joint modeling of recurrent event processes and intermittently observed time-varying binary covariate processes. *Lifetime data analysis*, 22(1):145–160, 2016.

[60] Dimitris Rizopoulos. Jm: An R package for the joint modelling of longitudinal and time-to-event data. *Journal of statistical software (Online)*, 35(9):1–33, 2010.

[61] Dimitris Rizopoulos. The R package jmbayes for fitting joint models for longitudinal and time-to-event data using mcmc. *arXiv preprint arXiv:1404.7625*, 2014.

[62] Pete Philipson, Peter Diggle, Ines Sousa, Ruwanthi Kolamunnage-Dona, Paula Williamson, and Robin Henderson. joiner: Joint modelling of repeated measurements and time-to-event data. 2012.

[63] Cécile Proust-Lima and Benoit Liquet. Lcmm: an R package for estimation of latent class mixed models and joint latent class models. In *The R User Conference, useR! 2011 August 16-18 2011 University of Warwick, Coventry, UK*, page 66. Citeseer, 2011.

[64] Menggang Yu, Ngayee J Law, Jeremy MG Taylor, and Howard M Sandler. Joint longitudinal-survival-cure models and their application to prostate cancer. *Statistica Sinica*, pages 835–862, 2004.

[65] Anastasios A Tsiatis, Victor Degruttola, and Michael S Wulfsohn. Modeling the relationship of survival to longitudinal data measured with error. applications to survival and cd4 counts in patients with aids. *Journal of the american statistical association*, 90(429):27–37, 1995.

[66] Michael S Wulfsohn and Anastasios A Tsiatis. A joint model for survival and longitudinal data measured with error. *Biometrics*, pages 330–339, 1997.

[67] Geert Verbeke. Linear mixed models for longitudinal data. In *Linear mixed models in practice*, pages 63–153. Springer, 1997.

[68] Dimitris Rizopoulos, Geert Verbeke, and Geert Molenberghs. Shared parameter models under random effects misspecification. *Biometrika*, 95(1):63–74, 2008.

[69] Jose Pinheiro, Douglas Bates, Saikat DebRoy, Deepayan Sarkar, et al. Linear and nonlinear mixed effects models. *R package version*, 3:57, 2007.

[70] D Bates, M Maechler, and B Bolker. The lme4 package, uppercaseR package, version 2. 2007.

[71] Terry M Therneau and Thomas Lumley. Package survival. *Survival analysis published on CRAN*, 2:3, 2014.

[72] Jimin Ding and Jane-Ling Wang. Modeling longitudinal data with nonparametric multiplicative random effects jointly with survival data. *Biometrics*, 64(2):546–556, 2008.

[73] Elizabeth R Brown, Joseph G Ibrahim, and Victor DeGruttola. A flexible b-spline model for multiple longitudinal biomarkers and survival. *Biometrics*, 61(1):64–73, 2005.

[74] Stephanie Green, Jacqueline Benedetti, Angela Smith, and John Crowley. *Clinical trials in oncology*, volume 28. CRC press, 2012.

[75] John O'Quigley, Margaret Pepe, and Lloyd Fisher. Continual reassessment method: a practical design for phase 1 clinical trials in cancer. *Biometrics*, pages 33–48, 1990.

[76] Steven N Goodman, Marianna L Zahurak, and Steven Piantadosi. Some practical improvements in the continual reassessment method for phase i studies. *Statistics in medicine*, 14(11):1149–1161, 1995.

[77] S Piantadosi, JD Fisher, and S Grossman. Practical implementation of a modified continual reassessment method for dose-finding trials. *Cancer chemotherapy and pharmacology*, 41(6):429–436, 1998.

[78] Z Yuan, R Chappell, and H Bailey. The continual reassessment method for multiple toxicity grades: a bayesian quasi-likelihood approach. *Biometrics*, 63(1):173–179, 2007.

[79] Ying Kuen Cheung and Rick Chappell. Sequential designs for phase I clinical trials with late-onset toxicities. *Biometrics*, 56(4):1177–1182, 2000.

[80] James Babb, André Rogatko, and Shelemyahu Zacks. Cancer phase-I clinical trials: efficient dose escalation with overdose control. *Statistics in medicine*, 17(10):1103–1120, 1998.

[81] André Rogatko, David Schoeneck, William Jonas, Mourad Tighiouart, Fadlo R Khuri, and Alan Porter. Translation of innovative designs into phase- uppercaseI trials. *Journal of clinical oncology*, 25(31):4982–4986, 2007.

[82] Ying Yuan, Beibei Guo, Mark Munsell, Karen Lu, and Amir Jazaeri. Midas: a practical bayesian design for platform trials with molecularly targeted agents. *Statistics in medicine*, 35(22):3892–3906, 2016.

[83] Victor Moreno García, David Olmos, Carlos Gomez-Roca, Philippe A Cassier, Rafael Morales-Barrera, Gianluca Del Conte, Elisa Gallerani, Andre T Brunetto, Patrick Schöffski, Silvia Marsoni, et al. Dose–response relationship in phase I clinical trials: a european drug development network (eddn) collaboration study. *Clinical cancer research*, 20(22):5663–5671, 2014.

[84] Stephen A Cannistra. Challenges and pitfalls of combining targeted agents in phase I studies, 2008.

[85] Wendy R Parulekar and Elizabeth A Eisenhauer. Phase I trial design for solid tumor studies of targeted, non-cytotoxic agents: theory and practice. *Journal of the national cancer institute*, 96(13):990–997, 2004.

[86] Edward L Korn, Susan G Arbuck, James M Pluda, Richard Simon, Richard S Kaplan, and Michaele C Christian. Clinical trial designs for cytostatic agents: are new approaches needed? *Journal of clinical oncology*, 19(1):265–272, 2001.

[87] Feifei Li, Changqi Zhao, and Lili Wang. Molecular-targeted agents combination therapy for cancer: developments and potentials. *International journal of cancer*, 134(6):1257–1269, 2014.

[88] J-C Soria, JY Blay, JP Spano, X Pivot, Y Coscas, and D Khayat. Added value of molecular targeted agents in oncology. *Annals of oncology*, 22(8):1703–1716, 2011.

[89] Sumithra J Mandrekar, Yue Cui, and Daniel J Sargent. An adaptive phase uppercaseI design for identifying a biologically optimal dose for dual agent drug combinations. *Statistics in medicine*, 26(11):2317–2330, 2007.

[90] Akihiro Hirakawa. An adaptive dose-finding approach for correlated bivariate binary and continuous outcomes in phase I oncology trials. *Statistics in medicine*, 31(6):516–532, 2012.

[91] Chunyan Cai, Ying Yuan, and Yuan Ji. A bayesian dose finding design for oncology clinical trials of combinational biological agents. *Journal of the royal statistical society: series C (applied statistics)*, 63(1):159–173, 2014.

[92] David B Dunson and Brian Neelon. Bayesian inference on order-constrained parameters in generalized linear models. *Biometrics*, 59(2):286–295, 2003.

[93] Laura H Gunn and David B Dunson. A transformation approach for incorporating monotone or unimodal constraints. *Biostatistics*, 6(3):434–449, 2005.

[94] Yisheng Li, B Nebiyou Bekele, Yuan Ji, and John D Cook. Dose-schedule finding in phase uppercaseI/IIclinical trials using a bayesian isotonic transformation. *Statistics in medicine*, 27(24):4895–4913, 2008.

[95] Ikuko Funatogawa, Takashi Funatogawa, and Yasuo Ohashi. An autoregressive linear mixed effects model for the analysis of longitudinal data which show profiles approaching asymptotes. *Statistics in medicine*, 26(9):2113–2130, 2007.

[96] Xu Xu, Min Yuan, and Partha Nandy. Analysis of dose–response in flexible dose titration clinical studies. *Pharmaceutical statistics*, 11(4):280–286, 2012.

[97] Toshihiro Misumi and Sadanori Konishi. Mixed effects historical varying-coefficient model for evaluating dose–response in flexible dose trials. *Journal of the royal statistical society: series C (applied statistics)*, 65(2):331–344, 2016.

[98] JQ Shi, B Wang, EJ Will, and RM West. Mixed-effects gaussian process functional regression models with application to dose–response curve prediction. *Statistics in medicine*, 31(26):3165–3177, 2012.

[99] Damla Şentürk and Hans-Georg Müller. Functional varying coefficient models for longitudinal data. *Journal of the american statistical association*, 105(491):1256–1264, 2010.

[100] Trevor Hastie and Robert Tibshirani. Varying-coefficient models. *Journal of the royal statistical society: series B (methodological)*, 55(4):757–779, 1993.

[101] Wensheng Guo. Functional mixed effects models. *Biometrics*, 58(1):121–128, 2002.

[102] Jian Qing Shi and Taeryon Choi. *Gaussian process regression analysis for functional data*. CRC Press, 2011.

[103] Hulin Wu and Jin-Ting Zhang. *Nonparametric regression methods for longitudinal data analysis: mixed-effects modeling approaches*, volume 515. John Wiley & Sons, 2006.

[104] Harvey Goldstein. Efficient statistical modelling of longitudinal data. *Annals of human biology*, 13(2):129–141, 1986.

[105] Nan M Laird and James H Ware. Random-effects models for longitudinal data. *Biometrics*, pages 963–974, 1982.

[106] Douglas Bates, Martin Mächler, Ben Bolker, and Steve Walker. Fitting linear mixed-effects models using lme4. *arXiv preprint arXiv:1406.5823*, 2014.

[107] Jose Pinheiro, Douglas Bates, Saikat DebRoy, Deepayan Sarkar, and R Core Team. nlme: Linear and nonlinear mixed effects models. *R package version*, 3(2), 2015.

[108] Elena N Naumova, Aviva Must, and Nan M Laird. Tutorial in biostatistics: evaluating the impact of critical periods in longitudinal studies of growth using piecewise mixed effects models. *International journal of epidemiology*, 30(6):1332–1341, 2001.

[109] Thomas M Braun, Zheng Yuan, and Peter F Thall. Determining a maximum-tolerated schedule of a cytotoxic agent. *Biometrics,* 61(2):335–343, 2005.

[110] Changying A Liu and Thomas M Braun. Parametric non-mixture cure models for schedule finding of therapeutic agents. *Journal of the Royal Statistical Society: Series C (Applied Statistics),* 58(2):225–236, 2009.

[111] Youyi Fong, Håvard Rue, and Jon Wakefield. Bayesian inference for generalized linear mixed models. *Biostatistics,* 11(3):397–412, 2010.

[112] Jarrod D Hadfield et al. Mcmc methods for multi-response generalized linear mixed models: the mcmcglmm r package. *Journal of statistical software,* 33(2):1–22, 2010.

[113] Bob Carpenter, Andrew Gelman, Matthew D Hoffman, Daniel Lee, Ben Goodrich, Michael Betancourt, Marcus Brubaker, Jiqiang Guo, Peter Li, and Allen Riddell. Stan: A probabilistic programming language. *Journal of statistical software,* 76(1), 2017.

[114] Andrew Gelman et al. Prior distributions for variance parameters in hierarchical models (comment on article by browne and draper). *Bayesian analysis,* 1(3):515–534, 2006.

[115] David J Lunn, Andrew Thomas, Nicky Best, and David Spiegelhalter. Winbugs-a bayesian modelling framework: concepts, structure, and extensibility. *Statistics and computing,* 10(4):325–337, 2000.

[116] Martyn Plummer. Jags: Just another gibbs sampler, 2004.

[117] Paul C Lambert, Alex J Sutton, Paul R Burton, Keith R Abrams, and David R Jones. How vague is vague? a simulation study of the impact of the use of vague prior distributions in mcmc using winbugs. *Statistics in medicine,* 24(15):2401–2428, 2005.

[118] Radford M Neal et al. Mcmc using hamiltonian dynamics. *Handbook of Markov chain Monte Carlo,* 2(11):2, 2011.

[119] Simon Duane, Anthony D Kennedy, Brian J Pendleton, and Duncan Roweth. Hybrid monte carlo. *Physics letters B,* 195(2):216–222, 1987.

[120] Matthew D Hoffman and Andrew Gelman. The no-u-turn sampler: adaptively setting path lengths in hamiltonian monte carlo. *Journal of machine learning research,* 15(1):1593–1623, 2014.

[121] Irina Sousa Moreira, Pedro Alexandrino Fernandes, and Maria Joao Ramos. Vascular endothelial growth factor (vegf) inhibition-a critical review. *Anti-cancer agents in medicinal chemistry (formerly current medicinal chemistry-anti-cancer agents),* 7(2):223–245, 2007.

[122] Paul CD Johnson, Sarah JE Barry, Heather M Ferguson, and Pie Müller. Power analysis for generalized linear mixed models in ecology and evolution. *Methods in ecology and evolution*, 6(2):133–142, 2015.

[123] Julien GA Martin, Daniel H Nussey, Alastair J Wilson, and Denis Réale. Measuring individual differences in reaction norms in field and experimental studies: a power analysis of random regression models. *Methods in ecology and evolution*, 2(4):362–374, 2011.

[124] Xianggui Qu. Linear mixed-effects models using R: A step-by-step approach, 2014.

[125] Nicholas G Reich, Jessica A Myers, Daniel Obeng, Aaron M Milstone, and Trish M Perl. Empirical power and sample size calculations for cluster-randomized and cluster-randomized crossover studies. *PLoS one*, 7(4), 2012.

[126] Christophe Le Tourneau, J Jack Lee, and Lillian L Siu. Dose escalation methods in phase I cancer clinical trials. *JNCI: Journal of the national cancer institute*, 101(10):708–720, 2009.

[127] Wei Zhang, Daniel J Sargent, and Sumithra Mandrekar. An adaptive dose-finding design incorporating both toxicity and efficacy. *Statistics in medicine*, 25(14):2365–2383, 2006.

[128] Mei-Yin Polley and Ying Kuen Cheung. Two-stage designs for dose-finding trials with a biologic endpoint using stepwise tests. *Biometrics*, 64(1):232–241, 2008.

[129] Yong Zang, J Jack Lee, and Ying Yuan. Adaptive designs for identifying optimal biological dose for molecularly targeted agents. *Clinical trials*, 11(3):319–327, 2014.

[130] Fang-Zhen Shen, Jing Wang, Jun Liang, Kun Mu, Ji-Yuan Hou, and Yan-Tao Wang. Low-dose metronomic chemotherapy with cisplatin: can it suppress angiogenesis in h22 hepatocarcinoma cells? *International journal of experimental pathology*, 91(1):10–16, 2010.

[131] Atanu Bhattacharjee and Vijay M Patil. Determining an optimum biological dose of a metronomic chemotherapy. *Journal of data science*, 15(1):77–94, 2017.

[132] Atanu Bhattacharjee and Vijay M Patil. Time-dependent area under the roc curve for optimum biological dose detection. *Turkiye klinikleri journal of biostatistics*, 8(2), 2016.

[133] Yuval Shaked, Alessia Ciarrocchi, Marcela Franco, Christina R Lee, Shan Man, Alison M Cheung, Daniel J Hicklin, David Chaplin, F Stuart

Foster, Robert Benezra, et al. Therapy-induced acute recruitment of circulating endothelial progenitor cells to tumors. *Science*, 313(5794):1785–1787, 2006.

[134] Q-B Lu. Molecular reaction mechanisms of combination treatments of low-dose cisplatin with radiotherapy and photodynamic therapy. *Journal of medicinal chemistry*, 50(11):2601–2604, 2007.

[135] D Malka, V Boige, N Jacques, N Vimond, A Adenis, E Boucher, JY Pierga, T Conroy, B Chauffert, E François, et al. Clinical value of circulating endothelial cell levels in metastatic colorectal cancer patients treated with first-line chemotherapy and bevacizumab. *Annals of oncology*, 23(4):919–927, 2012.

[136] Adrian M Jubb, Adam J Oates, Scott Holden, and Hartmut Koeppen. Predicting benefit from anti-angiogenic agents in malignancy. *Nature reviews cancer*, 6(8):626–635, 2006.

[137] Rupal S Bhatt, Pankaj Seth, and Vikas P Sukhatme. Biomarkers for monitoring antiangiogenic therapy. *Clinical cancer research*, 13(2):777s–780s, 2007.

[138] Francesco Bertolini, Yuval Shaked, Patrizia Mancuso, and Robert S Kerbel. The multifaceted circulating endothelial cell in cancer: towards marker and target identification. *Nature reviews cancer*, 6(11):835–845, 2006.

[139] Josep L Carrasco and Lluis Jover. Estimating the generalized concordance correlation coefficient through variance components. *Biometrics*, 59(4):849–858, 2003.

[140] Jacob Cohen. Weighted kappa: nominal scale agreement provision for scaled disagreement or partial credit. *Psychological bulletin*, 70(4):213, 1968.

[141] Jacob Cohen. A coefficient of agreement for nominal scales. *Educational and psychological measurement*, 20(1):37–46, 1960.

[142] Allan Donner and John J Koval. The estimation of intraclass correlation in the analysis of family data. *Biometrics*, pages 19–25, 1980.

[143] Ying Guo and Amita K Manatunga. Nonparametric estimation of the concordance correlation coefficient under univariate censoring. *Biometrics*, 63(1):164–172, 2007.

[144] Huiman X Barnhart and John M Williamson. Modeling concordance correlation via gee to evaluate reproducibility. *Biometrics*, 57(3):931–940, 2001.

[145] S Duggirala, H Larsen, RW Taylor, S Hanson, and CB Nemeroff. Pmcid: Pmc1381327.

[146] I Lawrence and Kuei Lin. Assay validation using the concordance correlation coefficient. *Biometrics*, pages 599–604, 1992.

[147] I Lawrence and Kuei Lin. A concordance correlation coefficient to evaluate reproducibility. *Biometrics*, pages 255–268, 1989.

[148] Feng Liang, Rui Paulo, German Molina, Merlise A Clyde, and Jim O Berger. Mixtures of g priors for bayesian variable selection. *Journal of the american statistical association*, 103(481):410–423, 2008.

[149] Jeffrey N Rouder, Paul L Speckman, Dongchu Sun, Richard D Morey, and Geoffrey Iverson. Bayesian t tests for accepting and rejecting the null hypothesis. *Psychonomic bulletin & review*, 16(2):225–237, 2009.

[150] Jeffrey N Rouder, Richard D Morey, Paul L Speckman, and Jordan M Province. Default bayes factors for anova designs. *Journal of mathematical psychology*, 56(5):356–374, 2012.

[151] Ruud Wetzels, Don van Ravenzwaaij, and Eric-Jan Wagenmakers. Bayesian analysis. *The encyclopedia of clinical psychology*, pages 1–11, 2014.

[152] Josep L Carrasco, Lluis Jover, Tonya S King, and Vernon M Chinchilli. Comparison of concordance correlation coefficient estimating approaches with skewed data. *Journal of biopharmaceutical statistics*, 17(4):673–684, 2007.

[153] Tonya S King and Vernon M Chinchilli. A generalized concordance correlation coefficient for continuous and categorical data. *Statistics in medicine*, 20(14):2131–2147, 2001.

[154] Xinhua Liu, Yunling Du, Jeanne Teresi, and Deborah S Hasin. Concordance correlation in the measurements of time to event. *Statistics in medicine*, 24(9):1409–1420, 2005.

[155] Weining Zhao Robieson. On weighted kappa and concordance correlation coefficient. *Ph.D. thesis*, 2000.

[156] Rebecca M Turner, Rumana Z Omar, and Simon G Thompson. Constructing intervals for the intracluster correlation coefficient using bayesian modelling, and application in cluster randomized trials. *Statistics in medicine*, 25(9):1443–1456, 2006.

[157] Robert Tibshirani. Regression shrinkage and selection via the lasso. *Journal of the royal statistical society: series B (Methodological)*, 58(1):267–288, 1996.

[158] Robert Tibshirani. The lasso method for variable selection in the cox model. *Statistics in medicine*, 16(4):385–395, 1997.

[159] Jianqing Fan and Runze Li. Variable selection via nonconcave penalized likelihood and its oracle properties. *Journal of the american statistical Association*, 96(456):1348–1360, 2001.

[160] Jianqing Fan and Runze Li. Variable selection for cox's proportional hazards model and frailty model. *Annals of statistics*, pages 74–99, 2002.

[161] Hui Zou and Trevor Hastie. Regularization and variable selection via the elastic net. *Journal of the royal statistical society: series B (statistical methodology)*, 67(2):301–320, 2005.

[162] Emmanuel Candes, Terence Tao, et al. The dantzig selector: Statistical estimation when p is much larger than n. *The annals of statistics*, 35(6):2313–2351, 2007.

[163] Hemant Ishwaran, Udaya B Kogalur, Eugene H Blackstone, Michael S Lauer, et al. Random survival forests. *The annals of applied statistics*, 2(3):841–860, 2008.

[164] Pierre JM Verweij and Hans C Van Houwelingen. Cross-validation in survival analysis. *Statistics in medicine*, 12(24):2305–2314, 1993.

[165] Erika Graf, Claudia Schmoor, Willi Sauerbrei, and Martin Schumacher. Assessment and comparison of prognostic classification schemes for survival data. *Statistics in medicine*, 18(17-18):2529–2545, 1999.

[166] Pierre JM Verweij and Hans C Van Houwelingen. Penalized likelihood in cox regression. *Statistics in medicine*, 13(23-24):2427–2436, 1994.

[167] Hege M Bøvelstad, Ståle Nygård, Hege L Størvold, Magne Aldrin, Ørnulf Borgan, Arnoldo Frigessi, and Ole Christian Lingjærde. Predicting survival from microarray data—a comparative study. *Bioinformatics*, 23(16):2080–2087, 2007.

Index

3+3 design, 33

Aalen-Nelson estimator, 67
ACC, 21
Accelerated failure time, 105
Accelerated titration design, 32
ALC, 21
Altshuler estimator, 67
Area under the ROC curve (AUC), 33
Asymptotically, 20
Autoregressive, 186

Bayesian factor, 202
Bayesian frailty survival, 104
Bayesian model average, 75
Bayesian sample size calculation, 23
Bayeslongitudinal, 134
BayesX package, 105
Breslow estimator, 215
BVSNLP package, 215

Circulating endothelial cell, 48
Clinical trial, 18, 19
coda package, 105
Competing risk, 87
Competing risk plot, 89
Compound symmetry, 170
Comprehensive R archive network (CRAN), 6
Concordance correlation coefficient(CCC), 199
Conditonal probability, 78
Confidence interval, 204
Continual reassessment method (CRM), 34
coprimary package, 29

covariance, 169
covariance matrix, 41
Covariance pattern, 170
Coverage probability, 28
Cox proportional hazards, 213
Credible band, 76
CRTSize package, 29
CT scan, 199
Cumulative hazard rate function, 67
Cumulative incidence function, 89

Data science, 226
Diagnostics for Cox's PH model , 72
Diagnostics test, 197
DNA methylation expression, 209
Dose escalation step dose, 32
Dose selection algorithm, 51
Dose-limiting toxicities (DLTs), 32
Dose-limiting toxicities(DLTs), 189
DPpackage, 134
Dynamic linear mixed effect model, 186

Elastic-Net, 223
Equivalence trial, 26
EurosarcBayes package, 29

fields package, 105
First order, 170
Fixed effect model, 188
flexsurv package, 120
Frailty data analysis, 97
Frailty on recurrent events, 104

Gene expression omnibus, 154
General covariance structure, 170
Gibbs, 7
glm, 185

241

Hazard function, 65
Heterogeneous compound symmetry, 171
Heterogeneous first-order autoregressive, 171
Heterogeneous toeplitz, 171
Heterogeneous uncorrelated, 171
High dimensional data analysis, 210
HighDimOut package, 224
Highest posterior density (HPD), 20
Hypothesis, 14

JM package, 166
Joint modeling, 153
JZS prior, 202

K-fold cross-validation, 226
Kaplan-Meier estimator, 66

L1 penalty function, 210
LASSO, 210
Linear mixed effect, 188
lme4, 186
lmer, 185
Log-Rank, 13
Logistics model, 41
Longitudinal data, 169
Longitudinal data analysis, 131
longpower package, 29

Marginal posterior distribution, 19
Maximum partial likelihood, 69
Maximum tolerable dose (MTD), 32, 195
MCMC (Markov chain Monte Carlo), 7
MCMCglmm, 192
Median probability model (MPM), 216
Metronomic chemotheapy, 190
Metropolis, 7
Microarray, 209
Missing at random, 144
Missing at random (MAR), 41
Missing data analysis, 143
Missing not at random, 144

Mixed effect model, 187
Mixed-effect model, 169
Molecular targeted agents(MTA), 186
MRI, 199
Multivariate normal distribution, 171

Net survival, 111
Non-inferiority trial, 26
Non-shrinkage failure, 41

Oncology trial, 18, 32
OpenBUGS, 7
Optimum, 21
Optimum biological dose (OBD), 186
Overall survival, 131

Partial log-likelihood, 215
Penalized cox's regression, 223
Pharmacologically guided dose escalation(PGDE) design, 33
Phase I trial, 32
Phase II, 39
Piecewise Hazard, 118
Piecewise hazard, 118
Posterior credible interval, 28
Posterior distribution, 18
Posterior error rate, 23
Posterior inclusion probability, 216
Power, 19
Principal component analysis, 212
Prior distribution, 18
Product inverse moment (piMOM), 216
Product limit, 66
Product-moment (pMOM), 216
Proportional hazards, 215

QOL, 131
Quadratic logistic design, 52

R, 3
R packages, 3
R2BayesX package, 105
Random effect model, 188

RCTs, 14
Relative survival, 111, 120
Right censoring, 65
Risk, 19
Rule-based design, 32

Sample size, 14, 18
samplesizelogisticcasecontrol
        pacakge, 29
SIMR package, 194
spBayesSurv, 106
spBayesSurv package, 105
Superiority trial, 26
Surveillance, epidemiology and end
        results, 111
Survival, 18
Survival analysis, 13
survival package, 66, 105

Time course data, 173
Time-dependent survival model, 154
Time-to-event, 68
Toeplitz, 170
Toxicity profile testing, 48
Type-I error, 18
Type-II error, 18

Vascular endothelial cells (VECs),
        195

Wald score, 71
Wald statistics, 42
Walds test, 119